Bariatric
Meal Prep

COOKBOOK

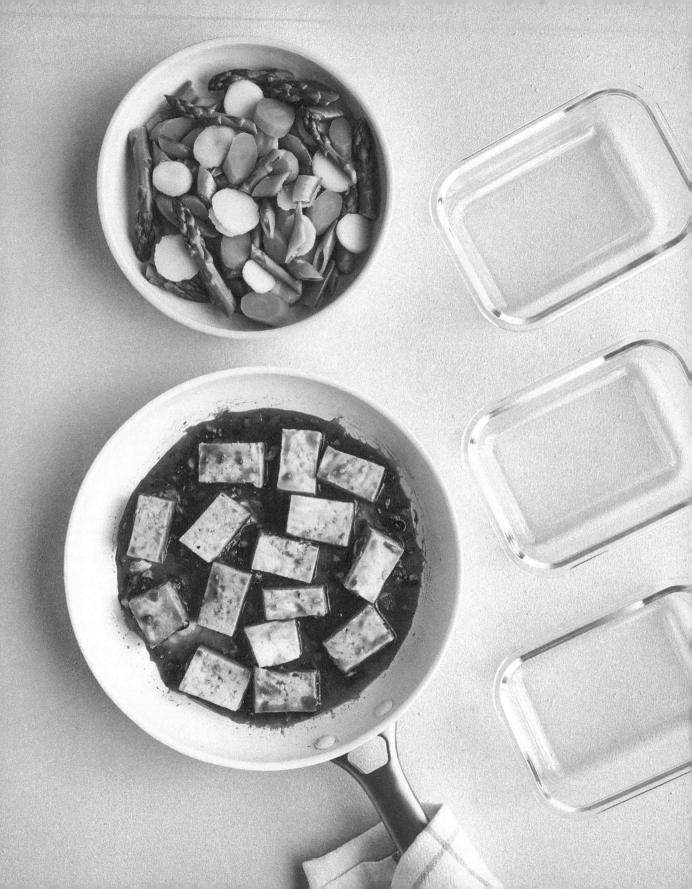

Bariatric Meal Prep

COOKBOOK

6 WEEKS of Perfectly Portioned Meals for Lifelong Weight Management

Andrea D'Oria, RD, CDN

Photography by Hélène Dujardin

ROCKRIDGE
PRESS

For general information on our other products and services or to obtain technical support, please contact our Customer Care Department within the United States at (866) 744-2665, or outside the United States at (510) 253-0500.

Rockridge Press publishes its books in a variety of electronic and print formats. Some content that appears in print may not be available in electronic books, and vice versa.

TRADEMARKS: Rockridge Press and the Rockridge Press logo are trademarks or registered trademarks of Callisto Media Inc. and/or its affiliates, in the United States and other countries, and may not be used without written permission. All other trademarks are the property of their respective owners. Rockridge Press is not associated with any product or vendor mentioned in this book.

Interior and Cover Designer: Richard Tapp
Art Producer: Sue Bischofberger
Editor: Anna Pulley
Production Editor: Andrew Yackira
Production Manager: Michael Kay

Photography © 2021 Hélène Dujardin, with food styling by Anna Hampton

Author photo courtesy of Dan Marino

ISBN: Print 978-1-64876-565-0
       eBook 978-1-64876-566-7

R0

To my boys, Daniel and Charles,
and my soul mate, Ron

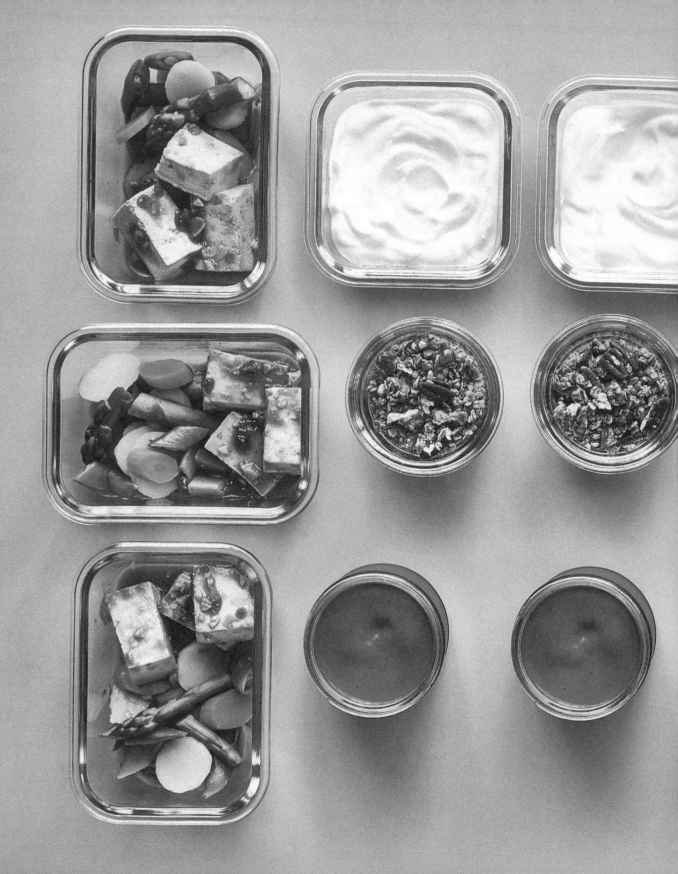

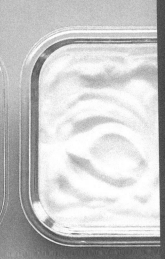
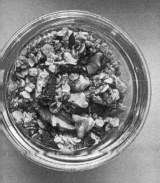
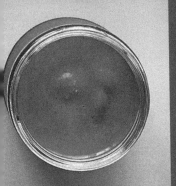

Contents

Introduction VIII

PART ONE: BARIATRIC MEAL PREP 1

Chapter One: Bariatric Eating and Lifestyle 3

Chapter Two: Bariatric Meal Prep Essentials 13

Chapter Three: Meal Preps for
Immediately Post-Surgery 25

Chapter Four: Meal Preps for General Diet 55

PART TWO: MORE RECIPES TO PREP 97

Chapter Five: Shakes, Smoothies,
and Breakfasts 99

Chapter Six: Soups and Stews 115

Chapter Seven: Healthy Mains 129

Chapter Eight: Sweets and Snacks 147

Measurement Conversions 160

Resources 161

References 162

Index 163

Introduction

I'd like to start by congratulating you on prioritizing your health. Whether you just decided to have bariatric surgery or have celebrated many "surgiversaries" already, I know you are committed. Surgery is a powerful tool for managing health, but it won't work if you don't. So, I am thrilled you took action and decided to incorporate meal prepping, too.

Whichever surgery you have had, gastric sleeve, bypass, duodenal switch, or LAP band, streamlining your meals and ensuring they are ready to go is a key factor in your long-term success. Last-minute decisions around food often hinder progress. This book will teach you how to set yourself up each week and take the guesswork out of your day. There is no better time than the present to develop a new routine.

I have benefited from meal prep many times in my life, especially when time was not on my side. Graduate school is when my meal prep journey started, 20 years ago. I was working full time while completing my master's degree in clinical nutrition at New York University. Buying two meals a day was not an option on my budget. Making dinner at 10 p.m. was also not an option. Meal prep helped considerably. After graduating I moved to Seattle, where I worked for five years as a research nutritionist. I was required to provide study participants with the tools needed to achieve a 10 percent weight loss goal in six months. One essential strategy I passed on included prepping meals ahead of time and tracking intake.

More than a decade later, I continued to pass on those same strategies as a bariatric nutritionist. Working with weight loss surgery patients for the last seven years taught me that the surgery alone does not guarantee long-term success. Planning and preparing are essential parts of the weight loss process, too.

One of the main advantages of meal prepping is that it helps you meet your protein goal consistently. It also reduces the time you spend cooking your meals, leaving you free to devote time to other areas of your life. And, of course, it prevents food waste. When you portion out the specific amount of food you need for each meal, you are less likely to throw out any unused food or leftovers.

This book walks you through the meal prep process step by step in order to eliminate the confusion and guesswork as you transition after surgery. It will assist you as you progress from a lifestyle where your meals were not a priority to one where every bite counts. There are six weeks of prep included here, plus an additional 35 recipes for you to create your own preps in the weeks to come. I promise you won't be limited to bland and boring diet recipes, either. You will find options to satisfy your need for comfort foods like pancakes, meat loaf, mashed potatoes, and even desserts like apple pie.

Sounds good enough for the whole family to enjoy, right? Because it is. The recipes work for anyone who would like to follow a healthy eating plan. So, regardless of where you are in your surgery journey, or how many people you are cooking for, let's roll up those sleeves and get this meal prep started.

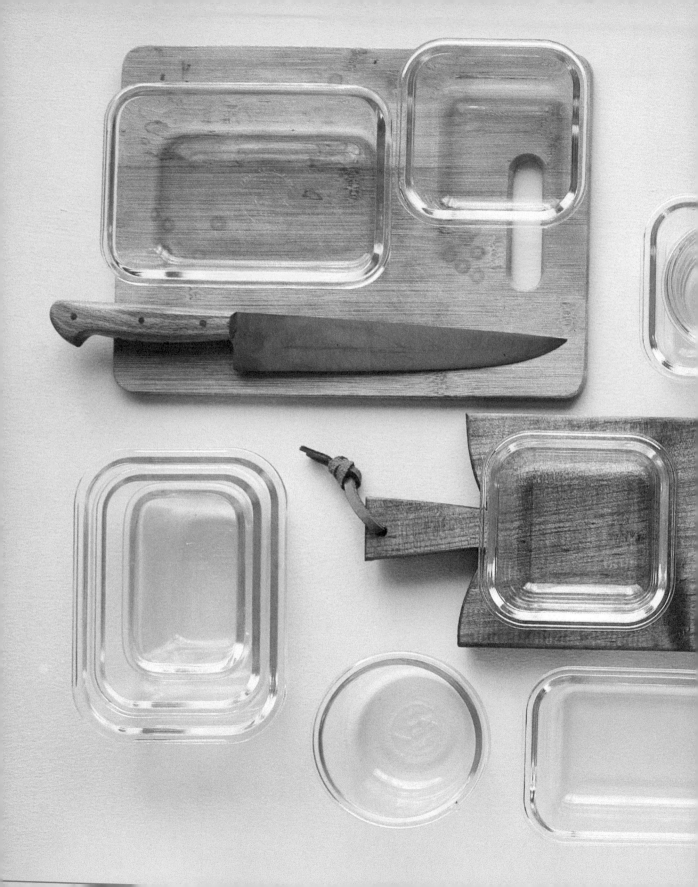

PART ONE

Bariatric Meal Prep

Following a bariatric diet is different from following any other diet you may have tried in the past; there are some unique challenges that only apply to those who have had a significant portion of their stomach surgically removed. This book is broken down into six meal prep sections based on the different diet phases (liquid, puree, soft, and general) that will help you recover from and thrive after bariatric surgery. Each section includes a shopping list, weekly meal grid, step-by-step instructions, and, of course, nutritious recipes. If you have not had your surgery yet, I recommend you get started early and begin storing and freezing mealtime necessities. This will help, because you will likely be tired and need to rest and recover after surgery. If you already had surgery, you might want to skip ahead to the general diet prep (meal preps 4 through 6), but you will still benefit from the information and recipes in the earlier phases.

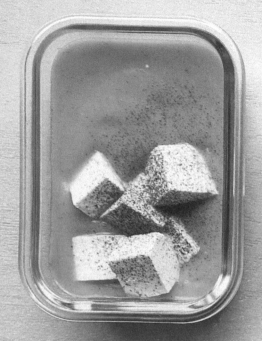

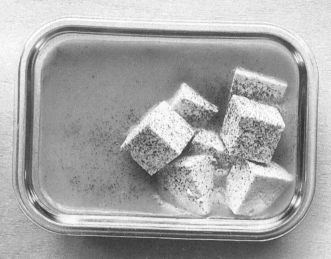

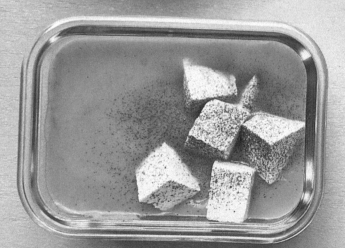

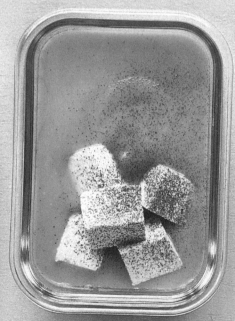

BUTTERNUT
SQUASH
SOUP **125**

CHAPTER ONE

Bariatric Eating and Lifestyle

Getting ready for surgery can bring on feelings of excitement and insecurity at the same time. You may feel overwhelmed if you have unanswered questions floating around in your head. However, you are already taking action and will find many of the answers you need in this book. Kudos to you on that.

I'd like you to let the fear go and the excitement flow. It's time to explore the many benefits of weight loss surgery and why it is essential to nourish your body for long-term success. Adjusting to your new bariatric lifestyle may take time, and you don't have to be perfect. But make a commitment to do your best. Keep in mind that eating meals with adequate protein, staying hydrated, and moving your body will keep you on the path toward a healthy post-surgery lifestyle that will last for years to come.

HAVING BARIATRIC SURGERY

Bariatric surgeries, like the gastric sleeve, bypass, and duodenal switch, are procedures that reduce the size of the stomach. Therefore, after one of these procedures, the volume of food that can be consumed at one time is limited. In some cases, there is also a reduction in the absorption of calories and certain nutrients. Ideally, your surgeon will explain the details of the procedures, and some may even offer videos you can watch of the actual surgery. (If you're squeamish I'd suggest you pass on that.)

You might be thinking that the smaller the stomach, the more weight you will lose after surgery. However, stomach size is not the sole component of significant weight loss after bariatric surgery. In fact, that factor is no longer considered a major contributor to long-term weight loss success.

Hormonal changes that occur in the top part of your stomach, a.k.a. the fundus, have been discovered to have a significant impact on your eating pattern and how you metabolize food. One such hormone is ghrelin, often referred to as the hunger hormone, which takes a dive after surgery. This drastic decrease means you will have little to no appetite. This affects how frequently and how much you will eat. Over time this hormone starts to rise, and you may notice your hunger starting again. The increase in appetite is not something to fear. I will address this concern in a later chapter and explain how to adapt so it does not negatively impact your results.

Rest assured that after you have undergone your bariatric procedure and read through this book, you will have the tools you need to lose a significant amount of weight and keep it off. According to a 2019 meta-analysis in the journal *Obesity Surgery*, most weight loss surgery patients achieve and maintain a loss of more than 50 percent of excess body weight over the long term.

Furthermore, the American Society for Metabolic and Bariatric Surgery (ASMBS) reports that bariatric surgery can lower the risk of death by as much as 40 percent, by helping to prevent and treat illnesses such as cancer, heart disease, and diabetes. I know it's hard to get excited about preventing health risks and things that may not even happen. So, let's talk about how surgery will impact your day-to-day life, too.

After surgery, most patients have better control of diabetes, high blood pressure, and reflux (heartburn), reducing the number of medications needed daily. Plus, the weight loss patients experience due to bariatric surgery can also improve obstructive sleep apnea (OSA), sometimes even eliminating the need to use a CPAP machine.

Having guided hundreds of patients through the early months after surgery, I know waiting for these results isn't easy. And there will be challenging moments. But I've seen firsthand how much better patients feel, physically and emotionally, and I can't wait for you to enjoy the fruits of your labor.

STAGES OF BARIATRIC EATING

Now that you have a thorough understanding of the benefits of surgery, let's get to the specifics of what bariatric eating looks like pre-surgery, post-surgery, and beyond. Your health care team should have provided you with specific guidelines to follow before and after surgery. It is crucial that you follow your doctor's orders. The nutrition and texture guidelines discussed in this section should supplement, not replace, the guidelines you are given.

Some bariatric programs have strict pre-op diets, limiting you to liquids only for two weeks, while others are more liberal, allowing you to include light meals. The same is true for when you transition from liquids to soft foods to solids. Remember, you are under your surgeon's care; you must follow your surgeon's recommendations. Progress through the following stages only as your medical provider clears you to do so.

Before Surgery: The Pre-Op Diet

The diet before surgery, which I'll refer to as pre-op, varies based on your surgeon. Therefore, there is no specific meal prep in the book for it. However, many bariatric programs require you to avoid solid food and simply drink liquids for 1 to 2 weeks, getting your calories and protein from shakes, broth, gelatins, ice pops, and so on. You can use the stage 1 meal preps in this book for suggestions, because they mirror a pre-op liquid diet.

Following a liquid diet may make you feel uneasy, which is understandable. I have yet to meet anyone who prefers to drink all their meals for weeks. However, I can't emphasize enough how much preparing your liquids ahead of time will help. The simple fact that you won't have to go into the grocery store and wander the aisles, seeing and smelling some of your favorite foods, will decrease temptation and cravings.

The pre-op liquid diet will help prepare you mentally for those first few weeks after surgery. It is good practice even if your surgeon does not require it for physical reasons, like pre-op weight loss or to reduce the size of your liver. Some of my patients have practiced eating only liquids for a few days each month before surgery while they are doing their six-month workup. It gave them an opportunity to try different recipes and protein shake combinations as well.

Stage 1: Liquid Diet

After you have undergone bariatric surgery, the next phase, meal prep 1 (page 26), is to focus on drinking for hydration and healing. One of the biggest concerns after you are discharged from the hospital is dehydration. And unlike surgeries to other areas of your body, bariatric surgery presents a direct obstacle, swelling, that will limit your stomach's capacity to hold essential liquids. I encourage you to pace yourself during the day and sip your clear liquids slowly. Clear liquids include water, broth, ice pops, and gelatins.

Once your surgeon gives you the go-ahead to include full liquids in your diet, often between day 3 and 7 post-op, reintroduce the protein powders and shakes. Your body needs protein to heal, so these shakes are not optional. The ones that tasted delicious to you before your surgery may no longer appeal to you. The taste of real sugar or artificial sweeteners may be unsettling, possibly even nauseating. For this reason, when reintroducing flavored beverages, diluting them with plain water or even milk first can be helpful.

As I mentioned, your body needs a minimum amount of protein each day. Protein is comprised of essential amino acids, which allows you to perform important body functions, like healing and providing you with energy. Your bariatric team will give you a specific protein goal to work toward. Initially after surgery, I encourage aiming for a minimum of 65 grams per day. It may take a little time to work up to, but stay focused. This meal prep plan is designed specifically to ensure that you hit the minimum daily protein goal of 65 grams. Of course, you will need more energy (calories) than that to function and recover, so the recipes contain some nutrient-dense carbohydrates and heart-healthy fats, too. Most patients cannot physically consume more than 600 calories, and some surgeons limit carbohydrates to under 40 grams. This would mean that your fat intake would need to be around 20 grams. However, I do not recommend you focus or track all macros at this early stage of recovery, as that can be stressful. Just focus on your protein.

Stage 2: Puree Diet

This is the stage that most patients report difficulty with. Reverting to a texture that reminds many people of baby food is hard. You may be tempted to advance to stage 3 ahead of schedule, but don't. Even if you are thinking you will chew it down to that puree texture, I caution you against it. The time line is for your safety; the incision needs to heal.

Stage 2 typically begins 8 to 14 days after surgery; in this book, it is meal prep 2 (page 33). If you are still working on reaching the minimum 65 grams of protein, this stage should help you get there. Pureeing food allows you to increase the protein density of your meals and snacks. And on the plus side, you get some much-needed mouthfeel and greater variety of flavors. I've had a few patients even tell me the first bite of hummus was heavenly.

You can also get creative and blend up protein-rich foods, like beans, tofu, cottage cheese, yogurt, and even fish. Meat is an option, too, although I have rarely had a patient who was willing to try pureed beef, pork, or poultry. You will see that I keep the recipes in this stage mostly vegetarian. These plant-based dishes provide fiber to help move food through your digestive tract and enable you to reach your nutrient goals. If you are tracking your intake on an app, don't be alarmed by the amount of carbs. You can still aim for the same macros from stage 1 (600 calories, 65 grams protein, 20 grams of carbohydrates, and 20 grams of fat). Again, these numbers may still be difficult to reach. Be sure to continue to keep your focus on protein first.

Stage 3: Soft Foods

The soft foods phase, meal prep 3, starts somewhere between 3 and 4 weeks post-op. This is a big milestone and one you may add to your calendar for a countdown. You will likely be more than ready to eat foods that require chewing during this stage. That said, it doesn't mean you have graduated to solid protein yet. I recommend using a quick fork test to determine if it is okay for you to eat the food. Take the back of a fork and press on the food. If the fork slides down to the plate and the food pushes through, it's soft enough to eat. For example, baked chicken breast and raw carrots are not *smashable*. Meat loaf and roasted carrots, on the other hand, pass the test.

Even though the food is soft in this phase, it's also crucial to remember the chewing part. I recommend that you aim to chew each bite 15 times, even if it is a food that seems like it can melt in your mouth. This slows you down and prevents you from overeating. When you eat more than your stomach can hold, it can be painful and cause vomiting. And although you will be including some carbohydrates in this phase, up to 50 grams, it should not be in the form of pasta, rice, or doughy breads. You can try to increase daily protein to 80 grams and slowly increase calories toward 800; this plan would give you about 30 grams for fat per day. It's important to work with your bariatric team, because capacity varies greatly among patients, and you are still in the healing stage.

Stage 4: General Diet

If your healing and recovery have gone well, you should be cleared to proceed with a healthy diet that includes all textures, meal preps 4 through 6, about 2 to 3 months after surgery. I often refer to this last phase as solid protein, because protein is still the primary macronutrient you'll focus on. Your tolerance will continue to improve as the months pass, so introduce new items in small amounts. Again, make sure you chew thoroughly, 15 to 20 times, before you swallow. You may find it takes a little longer to digest tough proteins, like shrimp, steak, and chicken breast, as well as foods that have thick skins, like apples and eggplants. I put those foods in the category of problem foods and will provide a more detailed list later. You can include some raw vegetables in this phase, too, like leafy greens.

In meal preps 4 and 5, most of the recipes ensure a higher moisture content, because you don't want to be eating dried-out food. Even if you chew them well, dry foods can feel like they won't exit your stomach; some of my patients described this as a "stuck" feeling, and it can lead to nausea and vomiting.

For at least the first year after your surgery, your attention needs to remain on protein. Over time it may be necessary to increase your daily protein goal from 75 to 80 grams, possibly up to 90 to 100 grams a day. Your calories will likely range from 800 to 1,000 a day as the year progresses, and they may increase after the first year, once you are in the maintenance phase. Speak with your bariatric program's nutritionist for your specific macro goals, because your specific nutrient goals will depend on your metrics (weight, height, age) and activity level.

GETTING ENOUGH WATER

Water is even more essential than protein; your body requires it for life-sustaining functions like waste removal and temperature regulation. Constipation and feeling cold are common complaints after surgery, and dehydration can enhance those issues, as well as dry skin, headaches, and fatigue. If you want to feel better faster after surgery, sip, sip, sip. The general rule of thumb is to aim for 64 ounces of caffeine-free fluid per day.

Fluids to reach for include water, caffeine-free tea, ice pops, broth, and even a half cup of decaf coffee. Don't drink carbonated beverages, like seltzer or diet soda, even if they are caffeine- and calorie-free. The gas in such beverages can cause unnecessary pain and discomfort.

Drinking too soon after your meal can cause pressure and gastrointestinal distress, so stay aware of the time. It is helpful to stop drinking 30 minutes before your meal and wait until 30 minutes after your meal to resume sipping. I would recommend practicing this drinking schedule as long as possible before surgery, starting with 5 to 10 minutes before and after meals.

Consider setting a timer after your meals, because your thirst signal may be muted. Then, work on sipping 16 ounces of water over a 2-hour period. Do this four times a day and you can get in the recommended 64 ounces. I call this technique *water blocking*. It would look something like this: 8 a.m. finish breakfast; 8:30 to 10:30 a.m. sip 16 ounces; 11:30 a.m. finish lunch; 12 to 2 p.m. sip 16 ounces.

HEALTHY LIVING

Once you've gone through the different post-surgery food phases, what do you need to know about the bariatric lifestyle and continued, sustained weight loss? The reduced stomach size and lessened hunger often mean you won't have to find ways to suppress the desire to eat in the early weeks and months after surgery. In addition, after bariatric surgery you'll feel fuller longer after eating. At times you may even need to remind yourself to eat.

If you're not used to eating on a schedule, this might prove difficult, but keep in mind that going long periods of time without eating is not the goal. Starvation and skipping meals put you at risk of malnutrition and hinder healthy, long-term weight loss success.

Healthy Eating Weeks, Months, and Years After Bariatric Surgery

Think of the first three months after surgery as a time to develop your nutrition foundation. Creating a habit of including lean protein in all your meals and snacks sets the tone for future choices. Including nutrient-dense vegetables and fruit also provides your body with much-needed vitamins and minerals. Together, the protein and essential nutrients nourish your body and give you the energy you need to complete your daily tasks, whether they involve taking care of family, working, or a mix of both. Preventing nutrient deficiencies can also help prevent cravings.

Staying consistent with shopping and prepping meals as the months pass ensures that taking care of your body becomes part of your normal routine. Plus, planning ahead decreases the temptation to return to pre-surgery habits, which can inhibit weight loss, especially because over time the hormone ghrelin will start to rise again and you will be able to tolerate larger portions. Sticking to your core choices and adjusting your meal preps to include slightly larger portions of lean protein and high-fiber vegetables will help keep you full and satisfied. The key to reducing the risk of regain is to keep your pattern consistent over time.

Keep an Eye on Nutrition and Macros

Eating protein-rich meals helps prevent potential complications from excessive muscle wasting. Therefore, tracking your macros is key. It doesn't need to be every day, however. I suggest you track your macros periodically. There are several websites and apps that can help you accomplish this. Start by working your way up to 20 to 30 grams of protein per meal. This will help you average between 60 and 90 grams per day without snacks.

It's also important to pick a protein powder that supports your goals. There are various different types of powders, and deciding between whey and plant-based protein options can be challenging. I recommend patients use whey if they are not experiencing any stomach issues, because whey is a complete protein that contains all the essential amino acids. Egg-based protein powders are also a good option. Collagen is often not as high in protein but mixes well and is versatile. You want to use a powder that has 20 to 30 grams of protein per serving. If you'd like to use plant-based protein powder, find one that includes a mix of ingredients (pea, hemp, soy) for a more complete protein.

It's helpful to have an unflavored protein powder on hand so you can use it in soups and other low-protein liquids. Also, read the directions on the packaging. (Some powders mix better in heated liquids without clumping.) Quick meal prep tip: Add protein powder to individual portions after reheating to help ensure even distribution and adequate intake per day.

Monitoring your intake of high-fat foods is extremely important as well. Too much fat in your meal will slow down digestion, indirectly reducing your protein intake. In addition, fat has the greatest number of calories per gram. So, just a few bites can quickly lead to excess calories and hinder weight loss.

You've probably been told to avoid fried foods. Frying is technically a dry-heat cooking method, but most of the time the oil is not hot enough, so the food soaks it up like a sponge. That's not the case in an air fryer, which you can use to get that crispy texture without all the oil.

Sugar should also be monitored closely. If you had bypass surgery, sugar can lead to dumping syndrome, causing sweating, cramps, nausea, and diarrhea. If you didn't have a bypass, limit sugar anyway. As you may have experienced before surgery, your intention to just have a little taste can "flip the switch," triggering a desire for more sugar. Be selective, check labels, and stick to snacks that have less than 10 grams of sugar per serving. Using sugar substitutes can also help avoid setbacks when your sweet tooth strikes; you'll see liquid stevia in some of the recipes.

Committing to an Exercise That Works

Once you are cleared to start exercising, get that body moving. Don't wait. Start slow, 10 to 15 minutes a day, and get the blood circulating. Choose movement that you enjoy, and avoid using exercise as a way to counter poor food choices.

Incorporate exercise into your daily routine to boost your mood, reduce stress, and get ahead of emotional eating. Exercise is also a great distraction technique if you find yourself snacking out of boredom. It releases endorphins and, most important, helps you sustain more muscle mass, which increases the calories your body burns.

The same as eating, I recommend setting a schedule each week to move your body, tracking your progress, whether that is steps or minutes, and treating yourself to a nonfood reward when you finish.

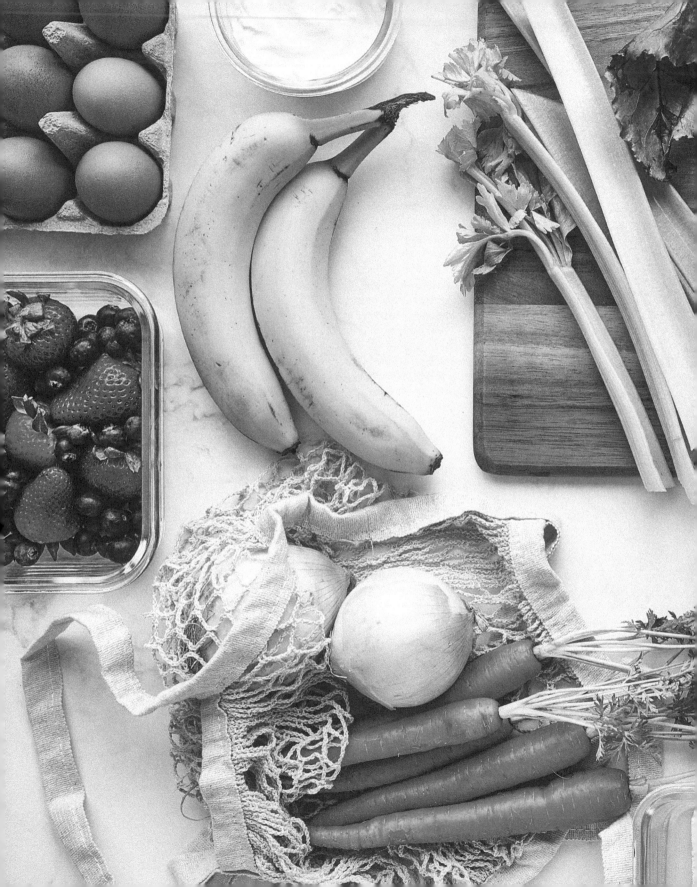

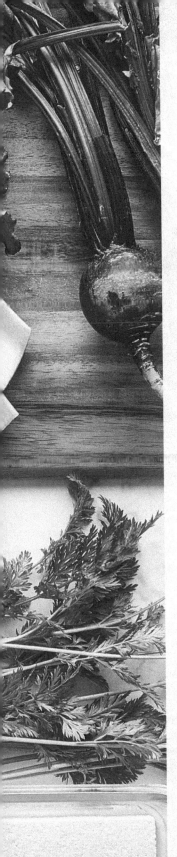

CHAPTER TWO

Bariatric Meal Prep Essentials

This chapter covers what meal prep is and why it's a great fit for people who've had bariatric surgery. Meal prepping involves spending one day (often on the weekend) prepping, cooking, and portioning balanced meals into containers for the whole week. The individual containers are important so you can grab them and go or heat up your meals easily at home.

Meal prepping works great with bariatric surgery because, while you may have the best intentions and a strong desire to turn your weight loss plan into reality, days are unpredictable and things get in the way. By having your meals prepped and ready to eat, you will take the guesswork out of eating and nourishing your body for the week.

WHY BARIATRIC MEAL PREP?

This new routine of eating may take time to adjust to, especially if you ate one meal a day before surgery. Eating five to six times a day will be necessary initially, but this doesn't mean taking that one meal and eating it again and again on the same day. You want some variety so you don't get bored of those essential high-quality proteins. For example, eggs and yogurt are two foods that tend to lose their appeal when eaten too frequently; this is something I'd like to prevent, given how valuable and versatile they are.

If cooking several different meals in a few hours sounds overwhelming, hang in there. We have a plan. In the next chapter you'll learn how to make bariatric-friendly meals and snacks for an entire week. The method is simple and easy and will offer variety. I promise it will be worth the initial discomfort that comes along with trying something new.

What makes meal prepping so handy? First, it is a time-saver. Having meals already made means you will not have to mess around in the kitchen, cooking and cleaning up every single day. Plus, your energy may peak and plummet at different points during the day. If you block off a few hours one day when you have the energy, you will increase your productivity. Later, when your energy is low, you won't be inclined to skip that meal and just sleep. Instead, you will recharge with your prepared meal, and maybe even add a workout once you are recharged.

Second, meal prep is cost-effective. You may have obligations that require you to change your schedule midweek or even midday. Meal prep ensures that the food you purchased will not spoil and end up in the garbage, a common complaint among those who have undergone bariatric surgery. When you plan to prep your meals all at once for the week ahead, you also shop more efficiently, purchasing items that are reused in multiple recipes and frozen foods that can be stored for months. Not to mention, portioning homemade meals into single servings is much cheaper than buying individually packaged premade meals, like Healthy Choice or Smart Ones, which are expensive and less nutritious.

Third, meal prep makes it easier to hit your numbers. I've designed these meals to help you achieve optimal portion control and appropriate macros, particularly protein, for each stage. If you decide to swap one meal for another at the end of one day, you won't need to make up for it later in the week. Just remember not to skip meals. Deficient nutrient intake will have a cumulative effect, perpetuating a cycle of low energy, poor choices, and a greater nutrient deficit. Unfortunately, I've seen this cycle happen many times in people who have undergone bariatric surgery, often ending with a trip to the hospital. Keep in mind that skipping meals is dangerous and not an option in the early months post-surgery.

What About Snacks?

The portions provided with each prep are suitable for your smaller, surgically altered stomach. The size of your meals and snacks will not vary greatly, nor will the nutrient profile. Snacks are sometimes referred to as mini meals and are meant to prevent you from going more than five hours without eating. Not eating for long periods of time can lead to fatigue, light-headedness, and low blood sugar.

I recommend having two to three snacks a day for the first few months after surgery. If you are an early riser and eat within two hours of waking up, you will likely need a mid-morning snack. For example, wake up at 6 a.m. and eat at 7 a.m., sip fluids from 8 to 10 a.m., and have your first snack at 10:30 a.m. Use the guideline of eating a small snack about 3½ to 4 hours after your meals. It may even be the three bites you could not finish at your previous meal. Meal preps 3 through 6 also include a snack option. At that stage, you may still be dividing a protein shake in half for your other snacks. Meal preps 1 and 2, the liquid and puree stages, provide three options and one snack per day. There are extra servings in the prep that you can add if you like. During those first stages, it will probably take a while to complete your meals, and you'll need to focus on drinking fluid in between. Your surgeon may also recommend a specific protein shake to include in your daily meal routine.

BENEFITS OF PRE-SURGERY PREP

If you are wondering when to start meal prepping, the answer is as soon as possible. Don't wait until after surgery. You will be tired, and you may not be able to focus as well. That's one reason why the first two meal preps are the simplest.

Getting yourself into the meal prep routine as early as possible will set you up for success. Like practicing the liquid diet, practicing prep prepares you mentally and helps you get into the swing of things. You might even start simply, prepping a few meals a week, to see what it's like.

I recommend doing the first two preps before surgery, perhaps stage 1 (liquids) on a Saturday and stage 2 (purees) on a Wednesday. You can't go wrong making the recipes for the early weeks of recovery well in advance, because they last a couple of months in the freezer. This will give you a few weeks after your surgery to rest and recover.

As you prepare and freeze the meals for the first stages of your new diet, keep in mind that the recipes in the early preps are intentionally mild in flavor. If you are tasting them before surgery and think something is missing, don't adjust the recipes just yet. After surgery, your sense of taste may be enhanced and you may even be sensitive to certain strong scents. Your preferences will likely vary, so resist the urge to create bolder flavors.

If you are inspired to stock up for later weeks, my suggestion is to get your soups on (see chapter 5). Soups freeze well, and you can even freeze some of them as ice cubes to add moisture to dishes or to defrost and sip during the first few days after surgery.

SIX-STEP PREP

Breaking any project down into smaller tasks makes it more manageable; that's why I encourage you to think of your preps as a system with six simple steps. No matter how simple the task seems, don't skip it—especially the first one.

Step 1: Choose Your Prep Day(s)

Start by designating a day of the week to get the preps done. Many people choose a weekend day, but do what works for your schedule. The preps will not take all day, usually just a few hours. And although it may not happen the same day each week, keeping this prep time as a weekly recurring "appointment" is useful.

Step 2: Make Your Plan

The first six preps are set for you, complete with shopping lists and meal charts, but it doesn't mean you can't enjoy some creativity. There will be items that you can swap in or out to better serve your taste preferences. For example, if you dislike peaches, you can replace them with mango or melon. There will also be bonus recipes you can incorporate from part 2, if you desire.

Step 3: Grocery Shop

It's important to recognize that shopping does not have to occur immediately before you meal prep. You can shop for the perishables on your grocery list a few days prior. You may need to adjust for freshness, so stay open-minded. The seasonality of certain produce items may limit availability or increase the cost, so if there's a deal at your grocery store or an in-season alternative, feel free to swap in other ingredients that make sense. (This is not the same as impulse purchases. A good rule of thumb is to limit yourself to three unplanned items per shopping trip.)

Step 4: Prepare and Cook

Organizing the items when you get home will help you be more efficient when you start cooking. Have designated areas in your pantry and refrigerator for more commonly used products, such as protein powder. Keep your measuring tools and storage containers together and easily accessible. Not having to search the kitchen drawers and cabinets will save time and stress.

Before you start cooking, get your ingredients out and lined up. Create a workstation. This will come in handy, because you will be doing a few different recipes in the same block of time and may need to bounce from one meal to the next. This is particularly helpful for the later preps that require more multitasking.

Step 5: Portion and Pack

Once your meals are cooked and cooled, you will need to make individual portions and pack them up. An important part of your bariatric meal prep is to store the meals in serving sizes suitable for one. Let's take a pot of Chicken and Cheddar Chili (page 59), for example. The recipe makes eight servings, so you will need eight storage containers. This will allow for quicker cooling and defrosting and ensure that you're getting the right portion sizes for each meal.

Step 6: Grab and Go

This is when you enjoy the fruits of your labor. Running out the door at the last minute or coming home exhausted will not get in the way of you hitting your nutrition goals. Just grab the meal(s) you need, reheat (if necessary), and enjoy. I can't tell you how many times clients shared that this was a lifesaver. Meal prep allows you to participate in last-minute events without worry.

ESSENTIAL EQUIPMENT

There are many cooking gadgets out there; however, there's no need to run out and spend hundreds of dollars on all-new equipment. You most likely already have the majority of essentials needed for the recipes in this book. The following are the absolute must-haves in the long run. Think of them as investments that will streamline your meal prep.

Baking sheet (12 by 18 inches). The larger size will allow you to cook enough for the whole week.

Chef's knife. The sharper the knife, the better, because the sharpened edge will give you more control when cutting tough proteins or hard vegetables. Misen and Wüsthof are good brands. If you can, get a set with an 8-inch knife and 3½-inch paring knife.

Cutting boards (plastic, flexible). Use separate boards for raw produce and meats. Plastic is easier to sanitize than wood is; food safety is of the utmost importance.

Fine-mesh strainer. The finer the mesh, the better. Try a three-piece set with insulated handles.

Food processor. This appliance is more versatile than a traditional blender, although you can stick with just a blender if you prefer. A food processor is great for creating stage 1 liquids and stage 2 purees. It can also be used to chop vegetables, grind nuts, and even mix up the ingredients for muffins and protein balls. If you don't have much room in the kitchen, you can pick up a mini (2.6-quart) model.

Funnel. You'll use this often when transferring liquids into small containers.

Ice cream scoop. Great for making equal-size portions.

Ice pop molds. You may prefer your liquids extremely cold, even in cold weather. You can transfer smoothie recipes into these molds for healthy homemade ice pops.

Peeler. Thick skins are hard to digest after surgery, so you'll want to remove them from fruits and vegetables.

Sauté pan or skillet with lid (12 inches). Look for one that can go from the stovetop directly into the oven.

Saucepans (1 quart and 2½ quart). Useful for cooking grains and making sauces and soups.

Scale. Getting accurate measurements of your ingredients will reduce recipe confusion. Dry and liquid measures vary, so weighing can help you avoid making mistakes. You will also get a more accurate calculation for your protein intake by weighing your portions after cooking.

Silicone liners and muffin cups. These are great for speeding up cleanup, especially when making muffins. However, parchment paper and cooking spray work just as well.

Slow cooker. This appliance is great for ensuring that your solid proteins turn out tender and moist. Although slow cooker recipes take a long time to complete, they are actually time-savers because you just set them and forget them.

Thermometer. Preventing foodborne illness is critical when you are recovering from surgery. If possible, purchase a digital instant-read thermometer. Checking your cooked food's temperature is a great habit to get into.

Whisk. Some dishes will separate when they thaw out and will need to be emulsified again.

Storage Containers

How you store your meals is essential for meal prep success. You don't have to purchase expensive storage containers, however. Some of my patients have found great deals at thrift stores and discount stores. That said, you want containers that will hold up in the dishwasher, freezer, and oven. Thicker, higher-quality glass and plastic containers are less likely to crack and break. Investing a little more up front means replacing fewer containers later on.

Because you will be storing at least three meals and one to two snacks each day for seven days, you will need at least 28 containers. You can supplement these with reusable storage bags for snacks or finger foods. You'll also want a variety of shapes and sizes with lids. Here are some options:

Single and multi-compartment: You will need more single-compartment containers initially, but a couple with two to three compartments can be helpful, too, because they allow you to store several meals in one container and save freezer/refrigerator space. Smaller containers are better for reducing the amount of air in your stored items, which affects freshness. Find containers that hold 4 to 6 ounces or jars that hold ½ or 1 cup of prepared meals. The more you can get with lock lids or twist tops the better. The rubber rim around the lid is a good indicator that it is leakproof and airtight. You will need a variety of glass and plastic containers as well for temperature compatibility.

Stackable/nestable: It's nice to have options that fit neatly together. This will help with organizing, and it will reduce the storage space you need for meal prepping.

Plastic: Look for BPA-free dishwasher- and microwave-safe containers. BPA is a chemical used in certain plastics that has been shown to leach into food when heated. Rectangular two-sided latch containers are airtight and leakproof. I recommend Rubbermaid and Snapware brands. You can even get kid-size tumblers with wire whisk shakers, which are great for smoothies.

Glass: Glass is preferable to plastic, because it is BPA-free and freezer-, microwave-, and dishwasher-friendly. You can find sets fitting the criteria mentioned above online. Simply search for homemade baby food storage sets. I recommend the 18-piece baby food set by Glasslock. Unlike the typical glass container combination sets, Glasslock's selection is better for numerous portion sizes. Ball's 4-ounce glass mason jars with plastic storage lids are great for shakes and soups, as well.

Overall, I would suggest starting with eight mason jars, eight small round containers, eight rectangular containers, four two-compartment containers, and four kid-size tumbler cups. Also, get some nontoxic reusable freezer bags, such as the RUSSBE snack-size or Stasher silicone bags that can be used for freezing and heating dishes.

LONG-TERM MEAL PREP SUCCESS FOR SUSTAINED WEIGHT LOSS

Meal prepping will not only save you time, money, and stress, but it will also prevent you from reverting to old habits and food choices that often lead to weight regain. So, let's review the principles that will allow you to conquer meal prep and achieve long-term success.

Batch Cooking

Imagine a week when you don't have to dirty your kitchen over and over again. Instead, you invest some time one day to make several dishes that you will store for the week or even weeks ahead. With batch cooking, you gather ingredients and cooking equipment, simultaneously cooking and cooling several servings at once. Then, you divide those recipes into perfectly portioned meals and snacks that will be at your disposal whenever it is time to eat. And the best part is you only need to clean up that messy kitchen once.

Reusing Ingredients

Reusing ingredients is great because it helps prevent waste and can be a real money saver. And protein-rich foods can be expensive. The preps in this book get creative with how you reuse your ingredients, seasoning your dishes differently so you don't end up with taste fatigue from eating the same dish three or even four days in a row. For example, with a couple of pounds of ground meat, you can make Italian meatballs, tacos, and sliders.

Know What to Freeze

To save time, prevent waste, and help sustain nutrients, it's important to freeze and store your food in individual servings. If you're storing past the week, wrap food in parchment paper and plastic wrap first to prevent air contact, which contributes to freezer burn. If you're storing liquid, leave a little room at the top for it to expand. Foods with a high water content, like cabbage and celery, often do not freeze well, because they wilt and become waterlogged after thawing. Milk-based items like cheese, sour cream, and cream sauces also fall into this category, because they tend to separate after freezing. Some recipes are better off left in the refrigerator to cool overnight first, because quick changes in temperature can sometimes affect the quality of reheated food, causing them to become rubbery or mushy; look for storage tips in the recipes for specific recommendations.

Learn the Best Ways to Reheat

For your meal prep to be a success, you want to ensure that the food you store retains its appeal when it is time to eat. No one wants to be stuck eating freezer-burned food or soggy, chewy dishes later. Because the way you reheat will make an impact on flavor and texture, you won't be putting all your dishes directly into the microwave before you eat them. (Although, food with a higher moisture content often reheats well that way.) Some recipes will be better if you thaw them first in the refrigerator, then lay them out evenly when reheating. You can also use the defrost function of your microwave, but check on it frequently, because small amounts around the edges of the food may start to cook on this setting. Some recipes may also call for using the same cooking method to reheat the food later.

PREPPING FOR ONE OR THE WHOLE FAMILY

The beauty of meal prep is that it can be done for one person or the whole family, simply by scaling up the recipes. Preps 1 through 3 are specific to the healing phase after surgery and designed for one person. However, meal preps 4 through 6 and the recipes in part 2 are versatile, healthy recipes that can be enjoyed by all family members.

Did you know that your entire family can benefit from your surgery? Well, they can if you get them on board with your meals. I can't tell you how many patients told me their family members were reaping the benefits of weight loss and lower cholesterol levels. Limiting the frequency with which you have to handle fried and high-sugar foods in the house also decreases temptation for you down the road. Avoid making different meals for everyone else, especially fried foods and starchy dishes, while you eat your lean protein and vegetables. Transition the whole family to this new lifestyle. This is the trickle-down effect.

The preps with six recipes will leave you with more meals than you can finish in a week. This is great, because you can rotate different meals in to decrease repetition and boredom. Not to mention, you can also cut down on the number of recipes you need to prep each week if you have been stocking up on the extra servings.

ABOUT THE RECIPES AND MEAL PREP PLANS

These meal preps are designed to transition you through all the stages after surgery. If it takes you a little longer to heal and progress than I've assumed it will for the purpose of this book, that will affect your ability to tolerate the next stage. Be sure to consult your medical team before advancing to a new phase. Being patient and waiting are signs of respect to your body. Being committed to your health means being committed to your own unique schedule.

The recipes are mostly limited to 10 ingredients, and the meal preps will provide structure and decrease confusion in the early months after surgery. If you are tired and uninterested in food, a common occurrence in the first few months after surgery, you can create an exact replica of the week provided. However, ultimately, the goal is to design your own meal plan for each week. Using the additional recipes in part 2 will allow you to add more variety and put your own personal touch on your plan.

Each prep includes a shopping list for the recipes you will make, a daily meal chart, and step-by-step instructions to teach you exactly how to prepare and cook each meal. Eventually, you will create a flow that works for you and, ideally, delegate some tasks if someone else is helping. The recipes also include specific instructions on how to store and reheat your individual portioned meals.

Variety is something you'll need as time passes. I strongly encourage you to try the recipes provided in part 2. You can even swap recipes in part 2 for ones in the meal preps, if you'd like. If a recipe from part 2 also works for stages 1 through 3 of the healing process, it'll be noted. Ready to get started?

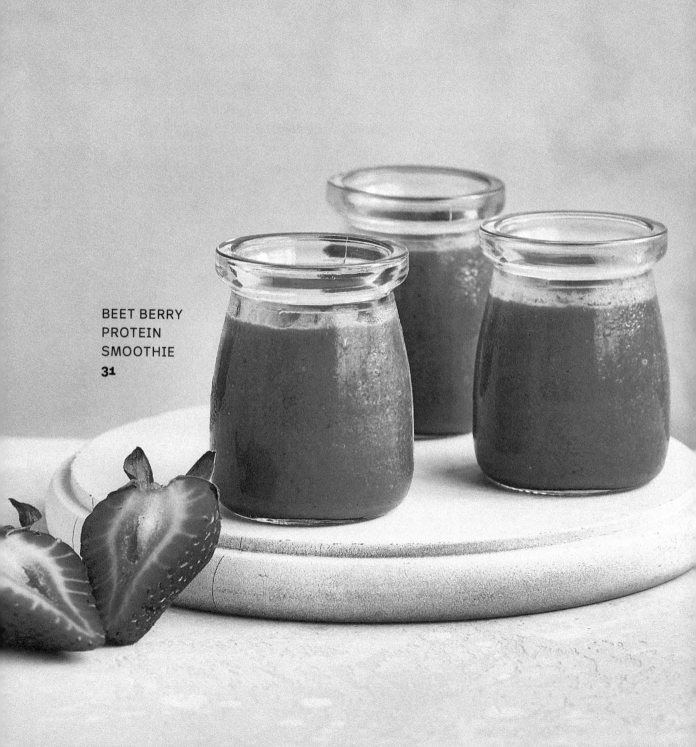

BEET BERRY
PROTEIN
SMOOTHIE
31

CHAPTER THREE

Meal Preps for Immediately Post-Surgery

This chapter will introduce the first three preps: liquid, puree, and soft food. Each will provide lists of ingredients, prep instructions, equipment, and storage containers you will need, plus recipes. There is also a chart that explains how to divide your meals throughout the week. Remember to consult with your bariatric surgeon or dietitian prior to introducing new foods or transitioning to the next stage.

The preps also include a guide for water intake. Do your best to sip throughout the day; it will get easier with each day that passes. Hydrating your body is a priority. Do not wait until you are thirsty. If you are using water to prepare your own protein shakes, do not count that toward your daily intake goal for clear liquids. If you are tracking your ounces each day using an app or website, tally your clear liquids separately.

PREP 1: STAGE 1, LIQUID DIET

The liquid diet includes both clear and full liquids. Clear liquids do not include protein and are limited to water, decaffeinated tea, gelatins, and clear broths. This prep includes clear liquids on day 1 only, because you will likely be at the hospital for the first two days after surgery, where they will provide you with your clear liquids. Start day 2 after you are cleared to include full liquids. Full liquids include milk, protein shakes, protein powders, and slightly thicker fluids like soups and smoothies. Introduce slowly; at first, you may want to limit your intake of full liquids to 2 ounces at a time. This liquid stage usually lasts 7 to 14 days, depending on your surgeon.

For week 1, keep the smoothies thinner, similar to a milk consistency. You may want to add more water, milk, or milk alternatives to thin them. As you move into week 2 and beyond, then you can reduce the liquid for a creamier, thicker texture. Remember that hydration is of the utmost importance these first few weeks. A saying I often use with my clients is, "fluid before food." Calories and protein will be low, which is to be expected, but dehydration must be prevented.

SHOPPING LIST

PRODUCE

- Bananas (5)
- Beets, small (2 to 3)
- Carrots (5 to 6)
- Celery stalks (4)
- Onion, large (1)
- Silken tofu, 1 (16-ounce) package

DAIRY AND DAIRY ALTERNATIVES

- Coconut milk, boxed, not canned (16 ounces)
- Greek yogurt, low-fat plain (8 ounces)
- Milk, low-fat, or higher-protein milk, such as Fairlife (16 ounces)

PROTEIN

- Eggs (12)
- Chicken drum-sticks (3 pounds)
- Protein powder, unflavored (16 scoops)

FROZEN

- Blueberries (16 ounces)
- Strawberries (16 ounces)

PANTRY/CANNED/BOTTLED

- Apple cider vinegar
- Bay leaves
- Black pepper, ground
- Chicken stock, low-sodium, 2 (32-ounce) boxes
- Cornstarch
- Ginger, ground
- Olive oil
- Sea salt
- Turmeric, ground

EQUIPMENT

- Baking sheet
- Blender/food processor
- Funnel
- Ladle
- Mixing bowl, large (1)
- Paring knife
- Saucepans, 2 (2¼-quart and 1-quart sizes)
- Slow cooker (6 quart)
- Storage containers, medium (16)
- Storage jars with lids (16)
- Strainer

	BREAKFAST	LUNCH	SNACK	DINNER	WATER
DAY 1	Bone Broth	Bone Broth	Egg Drop Soup	Egg Drop Soup	32 to 48 ounces
DAY 2	Beet Berry Protein Smoothie	Egg Drop Soup	Blueberry Tofu Smoothie	Bone Broth	32 to 48 ounces
DAY 3	Blueberry Tofu Smoothie	Bone Broth	Beet Berry Protein Smoothie	Egg Drop Soup	32 to 48 ounces
DAY 4	Blueberry Tofu Smoothie	Beet Berry Protein Smoothie	Egg Drop Soup	Bone Broth	32 to 48 ounces
DAY 5	Beet Berry Protein Smoothie	Bone Broth	Blueberry Tofu Smoothie	Egg Drop Soup	32 to 48 ounces
DAY 6	Blueberry Tofu Smoothie	Egg Drop Soup	Beet Berry Protein Smoothie	Bone Broth	32 to 48 ounces
DAY 7	Beet Berry Protein Smoothie	Bone Broth	Blueberry Tofu Smoothie	Egg Drop Soup	32 to 48 ounces

Step-by-Step Prep

1. Follow steps 1 and 2 in the Bone Broth recipe (page 29).

2. While the broth cooks, follow steps 1 and 2 in the Beet Berry Protein Smoothie recipe (page 31).

3. While the beets are roasting, follow steps 1 and 2 in the Egg Drop Soup recipe (page 30). Let the soup cool.

4. Make the Blueberry Tofu Smoothie (page 32) in its entirety.

5. Once the Egg Drop Soup is cool, finish the recipe and store.

6. Peel the beets and place them in the refrigerator. Once the beets are cold, follow steps 4 through 6 in the Beet Berry Protein Smoothie recipe.

7. Complete step 3 through 5 in the Bone Broth recipe.

Bone Broth

PREP TIME: 20 minutes / **COOK TIME:** 6 hours
MAKES 8 SERVINGS / GLUTEN-FREE, NUT-FREE, ONE POT

This bone broth is warm and soothing after surgery. It's loaded with key nutrients that help you heal, like calcium and magnesium. In addition, bone broth is rich in collagen and can aid in digestion. Don't let the cook time deter you. Once the prep is done, the slow cooker does all the work.

3 pounds chicken drumsticks or
  1 chicken carcass
5 carrots, chopped into large pieces
4 celery stalks, chopped into
  large pieces
1 onion, quartered
1 tablespoon apple cider vinegar

1 tablespoon sea salt (optional)
2 to 3 bay leaves
¼ teaspoon freshly ground black pepper
Water to cover, about 10 cups
8 scoops plain protein powder, divided
  (equal to 20 grams protein/serving)

1. In a 6-quart slow cooker, combine the chicken, carrots, celery, onion, vinegar, salt (if using), bay leaves, and pepper. Cover with the water.

2. Cover and cook on high heat for 6 hours or on low for 12 hours.

3. Once the broth is finished cooking, remove the meat from the bones; freeze the bones and meat in separate containers for future meals. Let the broth cool to room temperature, then strain the liquid and discard the solids.

4. Portion 1 cup of the cooled broth into each of 8 airtight containers and seal. If you plan to drink the broth as snacks, portion ½-cup servings.

5. Refrigerate the broth for up to 7 days. Freeze extra broth for up to 6 months.

6. To serve, reheat the broth, then add 1 scoop of protein powder to the warm (but not boiling) broth.

VARIATION: You can use 2 pounds of beef bone marrow in this recipe if you'd like. The marrow will provide more collagen.

PER SERVING: Calories: 15; Total fat: 0g; Total carbs: 1g; Sugar: 0g; Protein: 2g; Fiber: 0g; Sodium: 9mg

Egg Drop Soup

PREP TIME: 5 minutes / **COOK TIME:** 8 to 10 minutes

MAKES 8 SERVINGS / DAIRY-FREE, GLUTEN-FREE, NUT-FREE

This incredibly simple recipe is one of my patients' favorites. With this home-made option you can reduce the amount of sodium while enhancing its anti-inflammatory properties with ginger and turmeric. The ginger is a great addition, because it can help with nausea. However, if your taste buds are sensitive, reduce the amount by half.

6 cups chicken stock or Bone Broth (page 29)

½ teaspoon ground turmeric

¼ teaspoon ground ginger or ginger paste

1 tablespoon water

1 tablespoon cornstarch (omit if you prefer thinner soup)

1 tablespoon olive oil

⅛ teaspoon freshly ground black pepper

8 large eggs (optional, add to broth after you are cleared for full liquids)

1. In a large saucepan, combine the chicken stock, turmeric, and ginger over high heat; bring the mixture to a boil.

2. In a small bowl, mix the water and cornstarch (if using) with a fork to create a paste. Add the paste to the broth and continue to boil for 3 to 4 minutes to thicken the soup. Add the oil and pepper and stir. Set aside to cool.

3. Portion ¾ cup of soup into each of 8 airtight containers and seal.

4. Refrigerate 4 portions for up to 3 days, and freeze 4 portions for up to 4 months. Reheat individual servings in a small saucepan over medium heat.

5. To serve, beat 1 egg (if using) in a small bowl, and slowly pour it into the heated broth.

INGREDIENT TIP: Don't freeze the soup with the egg mixed in, because it will change the soup's texture. Reheat the broth from frozen before adding an egg, or skip the egg entirely and sip as a clear liquid.

PER SERVING: Calories: 37; Total fat: 2g; Total carbs: 2g; Sugar: 1g; Protein: 1g; Fiber: 0g; Sodium: 86mg

Beet Berry Protein Smoothie

PREP TIME: 10 minutes, plus 45 minutes to cool / **COOK TIME:** 1 hour

MAKES 8 SERVINGS / 5-INGREDIENT, GLUTEN-FREE, NUT-FREE, VEGETARIAN

This smoothie creates a beautiful vibrant color, as well as a sweet taste. The fuchsia, thanks to the beets, is stunning. Beet juice will stain, so be sure to avoid wearing anything you are not ready to part with. When peeling beets, do so over the sink and keep a bowl of water nearby to rinse your hands and utensils.

2 to 3 small beets

1 cup frozen strawberries

1½ cups low-fat or high-protein milk

1 cup low-fat plain Greek yogurt

1. Preheat the oven to 400°F.

2. Rinse the beets, trim the root and leaves (leaving about 1 inch of stem) and wrap the beets individually in aluminum foil.

3. Place on a baking sheet and roast for 1 hour. Insert the tip of a knife to test for tenderness. Allow to cool, until you can easily handle them.

4. Slowly open the foil and use foil, a paper towel, or disposable gloves to remove the skins. Cut off any remaining stem or root and chill in the refrigerator for 45 minutes.

5. Add the beets, berries, milk, and yogurt to a blender and blend until smooth. Add more milk for a thinner consistency.

6. Portion ½ cup of smoothie into each of 8 glass jars and seal.

7. Refrigerate 4 portions for up to 3 days, and freeze 4 portions for up to 2 months. Thaw frozen smoothies in the refrigerator overnight. Shake vigorously by hand prior before serving.

INGREDIENT TIP: If you're unaccustomed to the flavor of beets, decrease the amount to ½ cup and add ½ cup of strawberries. It is a mild flavor though, and roasting enhances the sweetness. To save time, purchase precooked beets; look for them in the prepared produce section of the grocery store.

PER SERVING: Calories: 55; Total fat: 1g; Total carbs: 9g; Sugar: 4g; Protein: 4g; Fiber: 1g; Sodium: 62mg

Blueberry Tofu Smoothie

PREP TIME: 10 minutes

MAKES 8 SERVINGS / 5-INGREDIENT, UNDER 10

Tofu is a great plant-based protein source that's easy to digest after surgery. It comes in different textures: soft or silken, firm, and extra-firm. Look for the soft or silken variety for shakes and pureeing to ensure the smoothness in your recipe.

6 ounces silken tofu

1½ cups frozen blueberries

1 frozen banana

2 cups coconut milk (boxed, not canned)

8 scoops plain protein powder (20 grams of protein per smoothie)

1. Drain the water from the tofu package.

2. In a blender, blend the tofu, blueberries, banana, and coconut milk until smooth. You may want to add a few drops of a liquid sugar substitute (such as stevia) depending on your taste preferences.

3. Portion ½ cup of smoothie into each of 8 resealable jars.

4. Refrigerate for up to 2 days or freeze for up to 2 months. Thaw frozen smoothies in the refrigerator overnight.

5. To serve, add the protein powder right before consuming the shake. Mix well with a shaker ball before sipping.

INGREDIENT TIP: This recipe makes great freezer pops, too. Be sure to thoroughly mix in the protein powder, then pour half of the liquid into ice pop molds and freeze until solid.

PER SERVING: Calories: 224; Total fat: 13g; Total carbs: 15g; Sugar: 5g; Protein: 14g; Fiber: 1g; Sodium: 84mg

PREP 2: STAGE 2, PUREE DIET

The pureed diet is an extension of the healing phase. It usually starts 8 to 15 days after surgery, when you still need to minimize friction along the incision line. Although not a favorite texture for most, the increased thickness in this stage will help you feel fuller after meals if you have been struggling with having an "empty feeling." The recipes here can be prepped before surgery, but you will need to freeze them to ensure that they stay fresh. This stage will also provide you with an opportunity to increase your protein, because the ingredients include more than dairy and protein powders. Keep in mind that this is still a spoon stage. Be sure that you blend each recipe to a smooth texture, strain when necessary, and avoid any chunks that require chewing.

SHOPPING LIST

PRODUCE

- Carrot, large (1)
- Cauliflower (1 large head)
- Garlic (1 head)

DAIRY

- Greek yogurt, low-fat plain (48 ounces)

PROTEIN

- Soft tofu (16 ounces)
- Protein powder, unflavored

FROZEN

- Peaches (8 ounces)

PANTRY/CANNED/BOTTLED

- Black pepper, ground
- Cumin, ground
- Flaxseed meal
- Garlic powder
- Lentils, red, dried
- Low-calorie liquid sweetener (such as stevia)

- Nonstick cooking spray
- Nutritional yeast
- Olive oil, extra-virgin
- Pumpkin pie spice
- Pumpkin puree, 1 (15-ounce) can
- Salt

- Turmeric, ground
- Vanilla extract
- Vegetable bouillon cube, low-sodium
- Vegetable broth (½ cup)

EQUIPMENT

- Baking sheet
- Food processor/blender
- Funnel
- Ladle
- Mixing bowl, large

- Paper towels
- Paring knife
- Roasting pan
- Saucepan (2.5 quart)

- Storage containers, medium (16)
- Storage jars with lids (16)
- Strainer
- Whisk

	BREAKFAST	LUNCH	DINNER	SNACK/DESSERT	WATER
DAY 1	Peach Parfait	Cauliflower Tofu Puree	Red Lentil Mash	Pumpkin Protein Pudding	48 to 56 ounces
DAY 2	Pumpkin Protein Pudding	Cauliflower Tofu Puree	Red Lentil Mash	Peach Parfait	48 to 56 ounces
DAY 3	Peach Parfait	Red Lentil Mash	Cauliflower Tofu Puree	Pumpkin Protein Pudding	48 to 56 ounces
DAY 4	Pumpkin Protein Pudding	Cauliflower Tofu Puree	Red Lentil Mash	Peach Parfait	48 to 56 ounces
DAY 5	Peach Parfait	Cauliflower Tofu Puree	Red Lentil Mash	Pumpkin Protein Pudding	48 to 56 ounces
DAY 6	Pumpkin Protein Pudding	Red Lentil Mash	Cauliflower Tofu Puree	Peach Parfait	48 to 56 ounces
DAY 7	Peach Parfait	Cauliflower Tofu Puree	Red Lentil Mash	Pumpkin Protein Pudding	48 to 56 ounces

Step-by-Step Prep

1. Follow steps 1 and 2 in the Cauliflower Tofu Puree recipe (page 36).

2. Next, complete steps 1 through 3 in the Red Lentil Mash recipe (page 38).

3. While that is simmering, make the Peach Parfait (page 39) to completion.

4. Check the Red Lentil Mash. If tender, remove from heat and let cool.

5. Get the tofu ready for the Cauliflower Tofu Puree; follow steps 3 and 4. Check the cauliflower; remove it from the heat if it is fork-tender.

6. Follow all the steps for the Pumpkin Protein Pudding recipe (page 40), including storage.

7. Divide and store the Red Lentil Mash.

8. Finish step 4 for the Cauliflower Tofu Puree.

Cauliflower Tofu Puree

PREP TIME: 30 minutes / **COOK TIME:** 45 minutes

MAKES 8 SERVINGS / GLUTEN-FREE, NUT-FREE

A great low-carb alternative to traditional mashed potatoes, this recipe is sure to be a favorite in the puree stage. After the healing process, use this as a side for codfish (page 143) or any of the chicken recipes in chapter 7 (page 129). You can increase the liquid with coconut milk and make a low-carb potato soup, as well. Nutritional yeast is very low in sodium and high in B vitamins, particularly vitamin B_{12}, which is why it's a great vegan substitute for grated cheese after bariatric surgery.

1 large head cauliflower

Nonstick cooking spray

3 tablespoons olive oil

¼ teaspoon salt

¼ teaspoon freshly ground black pepper

1 (8-ounce) package soft tofu

⅓ cup low-sodium vegetable broth

⅛ teaspoon garlic powder

8 scoops protein powder (20 grams per serving)

3 tablespoons nutritional yeast

1. Preheat the oven to 450°F.

2. Chop the cauliflower florets into even pieces. Spray a roasting pan with cooking spray and place the cauliflower in the pan. Drizzle the oil on the florets, and sprinkle with salt and pepper. Toss, spread evenly, and cook in the oven for about 40 minutes.

3. Drain the tofu and press gently between paper towels to remove additional liquid. In a food processor, combine the tofu, broth, garlic powder, and cooked cauliflower and blend well until smooth. Consistency should resemble mashed potatoes. Add more broth if needed.

4. Portion the puree evenly among 8 airtight containers, cool, and seal.

5. Refrigerate 4 containers for up to 4 days, and freeze 4 containers for up to 3 months. Reheat on the stove or in the microwave for 1 to 2 minutes.

6. To serve, whisk in the protein powder (chicken soup flavor works well) before enjoying and sprinkle with about 1 teaspoon of nutritional yeast.

PREP TIP: If you double this recipe, you can use it to replace the cauliflower in the Meat Loaf and Cauliflower Mash (page 47) in the next prep.

VARIATION: If you are not vegan, use Bone Broth (page 29) and grated Parmesan cheese in place of the vegetable broth and nutritional yeast.

PER SERVING: Calories: 159; Total fat: 7g; Total carbs: 7g; Sugar: 2g; Protein: 20g; Fiber: 3g; Sodium: 138mg

Red Lentil Mash

PREP TIME: 12 minutes / **COOK TIME:** 20 minutes

MAKES 8 SERVINGS / DAIRY-FREE, GLUTEN-FREE, VEGAN

Don't be concerned by the carbs here. Lentils provide 1 gram of protein for every 2 grams of carbohydrates. Mix in ¼ cup of plain Greek yogurt or cottage cheese for another 7 grams of protein.

1 tablespoon olive oil

4 garlic cloves, sliced

1 cup dry red lentils, rinsed

1 large carrot, chopped

½ teaspoon ground turmeric

½ teaspoon ground cumin

4 cups water

1 low-sodium vegetable bouillon cube

1. In a large saucepan, heat the oil on medium-low heat. Add the garlic and stir until slightly brown, about 1 minute.

2. Add the lentils, carrot, turmeric, and cumin. Stir and cook to release the aroma, about 2 minutes.

3. Add the water and bouillon, then increase the heat to high and bring to a boil. Once boiling, reduce the heat to low and simmer for about 20 minutes. The lentils will begin to fall apart when cooked.

4. Remove from the heat and let cool. Divide into small batches and pulse in a blender to create a thick liquid. (Strain to remove any pieces.)

5. Portion the lentils evenly among 8 airtight containers and seal.

6. Refrigerate 4 containers for up to 4 days, and freeze 4 containers for up to 6 months. To reheat from the refrigerator, microwave for 1 to 2 minutes. To reheat from frozen, thaw in the refrigerator overnight first. You can also heat directly from frozen in a saucepan by adding 1 to 2 tablespoons of water.

VARIATION: This recipe can easily be converted into a soup dish by adding Bone Broth (page 29) from prep 1 while heating.

PER SERVING (½ CUP): Calories: 110; Total fat: 2g; Total carbs: 17g; Sugar: 1g; Protein: 6g; Fiber: 3g; Sodium: 13mg

Peach Parfait

PREP TIME: 15 minutes

MAKES 8 SERVINGS / 5-INGREDIENT, GLUTEN-FREE, NUT-FREE, VEGETARIAN

Store-bought parfaits are often high in sugar, sometimes containing three to four times more sugar than recommended per meal or snack. This homemade option, however, is protein-packed and great for breakfast or dessert. You can easily replace the peach with other fruit, like mango. When you no longer have texture restrictions, skip the blending step and top with 1 tablespoon of chopped walnuts for a little more bite and some heart-healthy omega 3 fatty acids.

8 ounces frozen peaches

4 cups low-fat plain Greek yogurt

8 scoops plain protein powder
  (160 grams of protein)

1 tablespoon vanilla extract

3 tablespoons flaxseed meal

1. In a food processor or blender, puree the frozen peaches.

2. In a medium bowl, combine the yogurt, protein powder, and vanilla and mix well.

3. Portion ¼ cup of the yogurt mixture into each of 8 resealable jars. Then, add a layer of peach puree, about 2 tablespoons, followed by 1 teaspoon of flaxseed meal. Top with another layer of ¼ cup of yogurt and another layer of peach puree. Seal the jars tightly.

4. Refrigerate for up to 3 days or freeze for up to 1 week. If frozen, thaw overnight in the refrigerator before enjoying.

INGREDIENT TIP: If Greek yogurt is too thick for you at this stage, add milk, starting with 1 to 2 teaspoons at a time, and mix to the preferred texture.

PER SERVING: Calories: 179; Total fat: 3g; Total carbs: 18g; Sugar: 11g; Protein: 19g; Fiber: 1g; Sodium: 161mg

Pumpkin Protein Pudding

PREP TIME: 30 minutes

MAKES 8 SERVINGS / NUT-FREE, VEGETARIAN

Pumpkin is an excellent source of vitamin A, as well as vitamin C and many B vitamins. This recipe is low in sugar and a healthier alternative to store-bought puddings. Not to mention, the flavor sets it apart from the repetitiveness of chocolate and vanilla options. This recipe uses canned pumpkin to cut down on prep time; you can find it in the baking aisle with the pie fillings. Make sure you get pureed pumpkin, not pumpkin pie filling.

2 cups low-fat plain Greek yogurt

1 (15-ounce) can pumpkin puree

1 teaspoon pumpkin pie spice

1 teaspoon vanilla extract

Low-calorie sweetener, to taste (optional)

8 scoops plain protein powder (20 grams per serving)

1. In a large bowl, combine the yogurt, pumpkin, pumpkin pie spice, vanilla, and sweetener (if using); mix well.

2. Divide the pudding evenly among 8 airtight containers. Add protein powder into each serving and mix well. Seal the containers.

3. Refrigerate for up to 3 days or freeze up to 2 weeks. If frozen, thaw overnight in the refrigerator before enjoying.

VARIATION: For a dessert option, add 1 tablespoon of light whipped topping. If texture restrictions have been lifted, add 1 tablespoon of crumbled low-fat graham crackers, too.

PER SERVING: Calories: 129; Total fat: 1g; Total carbs: 10g; Sugar: 6g; Protein: 19g; Fiber: 2g; Sodium: 77mg

PREP 3: STAGE 3, SOFT DIET

It's finally time to enjoy food you can eat with a fork. This is a long-awaited moment for most. By now, you may even have a mental list of foods you want to eat again. You will return many of those foods to your diet in time, but I encourage you to move forward slowly.

Continuing to stick to the guidelines and choosing soft foods that provide your body with the macronutrients it needs is still the priority. This stage includes great sources of protein, such as fish, hard cheese, and ground meat. In addition, you can reintroduce soft vegetables and fruit (without thick skin).

Avoid foods that do not digest well, even though they are technically soft. Common problem foods include bread, pasta, rice, corn, leafy greens like spinach and Swiss chard, stringy vegetables like asparagus, cabbage, and fried foods. Continue to follow your surgeon's recommendations. If you are not sure about adding a certain item, then it is best to wait and speak with your medical team before introducing that food.

SHOPPING LIST

PRODUCE

- Apple (1)
- Bananas (4)
- Cauliflower (2 heads)
- Lemon (1)
- Onions, small (2)
- Spinach (1 [8-ounce] bag)
- Tomatoes, grape (1 pint)

DAIRY

- Feta cheese, reduced-fat, crumbled (5 ounces)
- Greek yogurt, low-fat plain (32 ounces)
- Milk, low-fat (16 ounces)
- Sour cream (¼ cup)

PROTEIN

- Eggs, 2 dozen
- Ground beef or ground turkey, lean (1½ pounds)
- Protein powder, unflavored (2 scoops)
- Protein powder, whey (½ cup)

FROZEN

- Salmon fillets (1 pound)

PANTRY/CANNED/BOTTLED

- Applesauce, unsweetened (½ cup)
- Baking soda
- Black pepper, ground
- Bread crumbs, Italian
- Bread crumbs, panko
- Cinnamon, ground
- Dijon mustard (optional)
- Dill, dried
- Flaxseed meal
- Flour, all-purpose
- Garlic powder
- Ketchup, no sugar added (optional)
- Mayonnaise, light
- Nonstick cooking spray
- Olive oil, extra-virgin
- Onion powder
- Onion soup mix, 1 packet
- Parmesan cheese, grated
- Parsley, dried
- Vanilla extract

EQUIPMENT

- Baking dish
- Baking sheet
- Food processor/ blender
- Paper towels
- Parchment paper or plastic wrap
- Paring knife
- Mixing bowls (3 large, 3 medium)
- Muffin tin and silicone liners
- Saucepan (2½-quart)
- Sauté pan or skillet
- Steamer basket
- Storage bags
- Storage containers: 16 medium, 8 dual-compartment
- Whisk

	BREAKFAST	LUNCH	DINNER	SNACK/DESSERT	WATER
DAY 1	Flourless Protein Pancakes	Meat Loaf and Cauliflower Mash	Salmon Cakes with Yogurt-Dill Sauce	Apple-Cinnamon Flax Muffins	56 to 64 ounces
DAY 2	Flourless Protein Pancakes	Meat Loaf and Cauliflower Mash	Salmon Cakes with Yogurt-Dill Sauce	Apple-Cinnamon Flax Muffins	56 to 64 ounces
DAY 3	Apple-Cinnamon Flax Muffins	Salmon Cakes with Yogurt-Dill Sauce	Meat Loaf and Cauliflower Mash	Flourless Protein Pancakes	56 to 64 ounces
DAY 4	Apple-Cinnamon Flax Muffins	Salmon Cakes with Yogurt-Dill Sauce	Meat Loaf and Cauliflower Mash	Flourless Protein Pancakes	56 to 64 ounces
DAY 5	Veggie Egg Cups	Salmon Cakes with Yogurt-Dill Sauce	Meat Loaf and Cauliflower Mash	Apple-Cinnamon Flax Muffins	56 to 64 ounces
DAY 6	Veggie Egg Cups	Flourless Protein Pancake	Salmon Cakes with Yogurt-Dill Sauce	Apple-Cinnamon Flax Muffins	56 to 64 ounces
DAY 7	Flourless Protein Pancakes	Veggie Egg Cups	Salmon Cakes with Yogurt-Dill Sauce	Meat Loaf Cauliflower Mash	56 to 64 ounces

Step-by-Step Prep

1. Complete steps 1 through 5 of the Salmon Cakes with Yogurt-Dill Sauce recipe (page 45). Set a timer for 10 minutes, then follow step 6 for the dill sauce. Set the salmon aside to cool.

2. Follow steps 1 through 5 of the Meat Loaf and Cauliflower Mash recipe (page 47). Place the meat loaf in the oven and set the timer for 1 hour. Steam the cauliflower, steps 6 and 7.

3. Complete steps 1 through 5 of the Veggie Egg Cups recipe (page 49) and place them in the oven with the meat loaf. Set a timer for 22 minutes.

4. Check the cauliflower; if it's fork-tender, remove it from the heat.

5. Complete steps 7 through 9 of the Salmon Cakes recipe.

6. Make the Flourless Protein Pancakes (page 50) to completion.

7. Prep steps 1 through 6 of the Apple-Cinnamon Flax Muffins recipe (page 51).

8. After the meat loaf has finished cooking, set a timer for 12 minutes, reduce the oven to 325°F, and bake the muffins.

9. Complete the Meat Loaf and Cauliflower Mash (steps 8 through 10).

10. Finish the Salmon Cakes and store.

11. Cool and store the Veggie Egg Cups and Apple Flax Muffins.

Salmon Cakes with Yogurt-Dill Sauce

PREP TIME: 15 minutes, plus 1 hour chill time / **COOK TIME:** 10 minutes
MAKES 8 SERVINGS / NUT-FREE

These flavorful salmon cakes make me feel like I'm out to brunch, and they make this great source of protein easy to digest. However, fish is a more expensive protein source, especially if you choose fresh. This recipe uses individually portioned frozen salmon, which is easier on your budget. Canned salmon and individual vacuum-sealed salmon packets can be substituted as well.

1 pound frozen salmon fillets, thawed

2 tablespoons olive oil

3 tablespoons lemon juice, divided

1 cup low-fat plain Greek yogurt

1 tablespoon Dijon mustard (optional)

½ teaspoon dried dill

¼ teaspoon freshly ground black pepper

½ cup panko bread crumbs

2 large eggs, beaten

2 tablespoons light mayonnaise

1 tablespoon dried parsley

1. Preheat the oven to 425°F.

2. Pat the thawed salmon fillets dry with a paper towel and place them on a parchment paper–lined baking sheet.

3. In a small bowl, mix the oil with 2 tablespoons of lemon juice, then brush this mixture on the fish.

4. Transfer the baking sheet to the oven and bake the salmon for 10 to 15 minutes, depending on thickness. The fish is done when it flakes easily with a fork and the color changes.

5. Let the salmon cool and rest for at least 10 minutes.

6. In a small bowl, mix together the remaining 1 tablespoon of lemon juice, yogurt, mustard (if using), dill, and pepper.

7. Using a fork, flake the salmon into small pieces and remove any bones.

continued

8. In a large bowl, combine the salmon, bread crumbs, eggs, mayonnaise, and parsley; mix well. Refrigerate for at least 1 hour.

9. Once the salmon mixture is cold, make 8 patties (2 to 3 ounces each). Reduce the oven to 375°F. Place the cakes on a baking sheet and bake for 20 minutes, flipping them halfway through. Remove the patties from the oven and let them cool.

10. Portion 1 salmon cake into each of 8 airtight containers and seal. Portion 2 to 3 tablespoons of sauce into each of 8 small airtight containers.

11. Refrigerate 4 of the salmon cakes for up to 4 days, and freeze the remaining 4 cakes for up to 2 months. Refrigerate the sauce for up to 1 week. (Don't freeze the sauce.) To reheat the salmon cakes from frozen, bake them at 375°F for 30 minutes, flipping them halfway through.

SERVING TIP: Ensure that the fish cake is not dry by adding some lemon juice and a little yogurt-dill sauce to each bite.

PER SERVING: Calories: 176; Total fat: 10g; Total carbs: 5g; Sugar: 3g; Protein: 15g; Fiber: 0g; Sodium: 119mg

Meat Loaf and Cauliflower Mash

PREP TIME: 25 minutes / **COOK TIME:** 1 hour
MAKES 8 SERVINGS / NUT-FREE

If you're craving comfort food, this meat loaf and mash will hit the spot. It's full of flavors that get better after being stored for a day or two, which is why this is great for meal prep. Beef is sometimes difficult to digest, due to its high fat content; look for 90/10 ground beef, which usually has about 10 grams of fat per 3-ounce serving. If there is no label, find beef that has a deeper red color. If you are concerned about the fat content or your tolerance, swap out the beef for extra-lean ground turkey or chicken. Look for less than 5 grams of fat per 3-ounce serving.

For the meat loaf

1½ pounds lean ground beef

1 onion, finely chopped

1 cup low-fat milk

1 cup dried Italian bread crumbs

1 large egg

½ packet onion soup mix

⅓ cup sugar-free ketchup, plus more for topping (optional)

For the mash

1 cauliflower head, cut into florets

¼ cup low-fat milk

¼ cup low-fat sour cream

¼ cup low-fat plain Greek yogurt

2 tablespoons grated Parmesan cheese

¼ teaspoon onion powder

To make the meat loaf

1. Preheat the oven to 350°F.

2. In a large bowl, combine the ground beef, onion, milk, bread crumbs, egg, onion soup mix, and ketchup (if using).

3. Form the mixture into a loaf shape and place it in a lightly greased baking dish.

4. Spread more ketchup (if using) on top to lightly coat the meat loaf.

5. Bake for 1 hour. Let cool, then cut into 8 portions.

continued

To make the mash

6. In a medium pot, bring 1 inch of water to a boil. Place the cauliflower in a steamer basket, lower the basket into the pot over the boiling water, and cover with a lid. Steam for 10 to 15 minutes, until fork-tender.

7. Place the steamed cauliflower in a food processor or blender. Pulse until the cauliflower is chopped into small pieces, then pour in the milk, sour cream, yogurt, cheese, and onion powder. Blend until smooth. If you prefer a thicker consistency, reduce the amount of milk and increase the amount of yogurt.

8. Portion the mash and meat loaf evenly into 8 airtight, dual-compartment containers.

9. Refrigerate 4 containers for up to 4 days, and freeze 4 containers for up to 2 months. To reheat the meat loaf and mash from frozen, remove the lid and top the container loosely with foil. Bake at 350°F for about 20 minutes.

PREP TIP: If you are using leftover cauliflower from stage 2's Cauliflower Tofu Puree (page 36), you will need to thicken the mash. Put it in a pan over low heat and let the water evaporate. Stirring in some low-fat cream cheese will also help create a thicker texture.

PER SERVING: Calories: 220; Total fat: 8g; Total carbs: 15g; Sugar: 5g; Protein: 24g; Fiber: 2g; Sodium: 298mg

Veggie Egg Cups

PREP TIME: 10 minutes / **COOK TIME:** 22 minutes

MAKES 12 CUPS / GLUTEN-FREE, NUT-FREE, VEGETARIAN

These cups are one of my most popular recipes for after weight loss surgery. You can use so many different ingredient combinations, including sautéed onions, spinach, mushroom, and Swiss; broccoli, cheddar, and diced ham; or zucchini, eggplant, tomato, and mozzarella. However, although you can experiment with different combinations, I do recommend you limit the use of processed meats like bacon and sausage, which are high in saturated fat, to once a week.

Nonstick cooking spray

12 large eggs

¼ cup low-fat milk

3 tablespoons minced onion

1 tablespoon garlic powder

1 (8-ounce) bag baby spinach

1 pint grape tomatoes

1 cup crumbled reduced-fat feta cheese

1. Preheat the oven to 350°F. Spray a 12-cup muffin tin with cooking spray.

2. In a large bowl, combine the eggs, milk, onion, and garlic powder. Mix well.

3. Divide the spinach, tomatoes, and feta among the muffin cups.

4. Pour the egg mixture evenly into each muffin cup. Bake for 22 to 25 minutes, until the egg mixture has set. Remove the cups from the muffin tin and let them cool completely.

5. Portion 1 egg cup into each of 12 storage bags or containers.

6. Refrigerate for up to 3 days or freeze for up to 2 months. Reheat in the microwave for 1 minute, adding 30 seconds if the center is still cool.

INGREDIENT TIP: One egg cup may be too large for one meal in your first month, depending on what you add to it. Stop eating at the first sign of fullness.

PER SERVING (1 EGG CUP): Calories: 109; Total fat: 7g; Total carbs: 3g; Sugar: 1g; Protein: 9g; Fiber: 1g; Sodium: 176mg

Flourless Protein Pancakes

PREP TIME: 5 minutes / **COOK TIME:** 10 minutes
MAKES 6 SERVINGS / GLUTEN-FREE, NUT-FREE, VEGETARIAN

Yes, you can have pancakes after weight loss surgery, but I am not referring to the sugar-soaked towers served at your local breakfast place. These pancakes are a delicious and nutritious option, and with just a few basic ingredients, you can make a whole week's worth in a short amount of time. Instead of enjoying these with syrup, add more protein. Top them with yogurt, smoked salmon, or even an over-easy egg on a day when you have more time. Think of these pancakes like open-faced breakfast sandwiches.

4 ripe bananas, mashed

6 large eggs

2 scoops unflavored protein powder
(40 grams of protein)

2 teaspoons vanilla extract

1 teaspoon ground cinnamon

Nonstick cooking spray

1. In a large bowl, combine the bananas, eggs, protein powder, vanilla, and cinnamon.

2. Heat a large pan over medium heat and spray it with cooking spray.

3. Spoon about ⅓ cup batter onto the skillet, cook until small bubbles form, 2 to 3 minutes, and then flip and cook for 2 to 3 minutes more. Repeat with the rest of the batter to make a total of 6 pancakes.

4. Portion 1 pancake into each of 6 resealable bags.

5. Refrigerate for up to 2 to 3 days or freeze for up to 2 months. If freezing, place a piece of parchment paper in between layers to prevent them from sticking together. Reheat in the toaster directly from the freezer.

VARIATION: You can also top these pancakes with fresh berries, nuts, and whipped cream.

PER SERVING: Calories: 170; Total fat: 5g; Total carbs: 19g; Sugar: 10g; Protein: 12g; Fiber: 3g; Sodium: 82mg

Apple-Cinnamon Flax Muffins

PREP TIME: 15 minutes / **COOK TIME:** 12 to 15 minutes
MAKES 12 MUFFINS / NUT-FREE

Muffins are great on the go, but store-bought options tend to be high in carbs and low in protein. Not these muffins. However, baking with protein powder can be tricky, because it can toughen the muffins. I use whey protein powder here; if you prefer a dairy-free powder, like pea or soy, here are a couple tips to keep in mind: Some brands do not recommend heating above 140°F, so read the label before purchasing. Use less protein powder than flour, and make sure that the recipe has enough moisture, because protein powder is absorbent.

Nonstick cooking spray
½ cup whey protein powder (40 to
  50 grams of protein)
½ cup all-purpose flour
1 teaspoon baking soda
½ teaspoon ground cinnamon

¼ cup flaxseed meal
¼ cup water
1½ cups unsweetened applesauce
1 large apple, cored, peeled, and
  chopped into small pieces
2 large eggs, beaten

1. Preheat the oven to 325°F. Spray a 12-cup muffin tin with cooking spray.

2. In a medium bowl, mix together the protein powder, flour, baking soda, and cinnamon.

3. In a separate medium bowl, whisk the flaxseed and water together, then add the applesauce, apple, and eggs.

4. Gently mix the dry ingredients into the wet ingredients, being careful not to overmix, because this will toughen the muffins. Divide the batter among the prepared muffin cups.

5. Cover with foil and bake for 6 minutes. (The foil helps hold in moisture and prevents the muffins from getting too brown on top.) Remove the foil and bake for 6 to 9 minutes more, until a knife or toothpick inserted in the center comes out clean. Let cool completely.

continued

6. Store in an airtight bag for 1 week on the countertop, or wrap the muffins individually with plastic wrap, place them in an airtight freezer bag, and freeze for up to 3 months. Reheat in an oven or toaster oven for 15 minutes at 375°F or microwave for 30 to 45 seconds.

INGREDIENT TIP: Top these with low-fat cream cheese, sugar-free jam, or home-made preserves.

PER SERVING: Calories: 78; Total fat: 2g; Total carbs: 12g; Sugar: 5g; Protein: 4g; Fiber: 2g; Sodium: 131mg

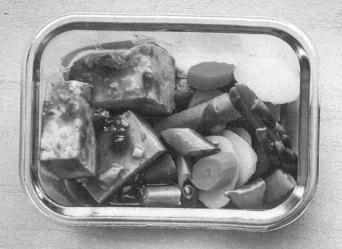

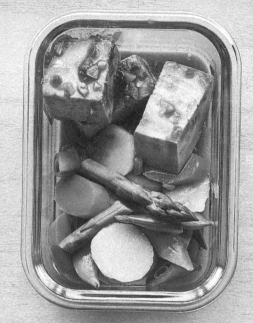

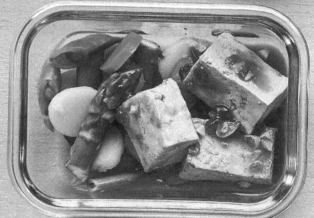

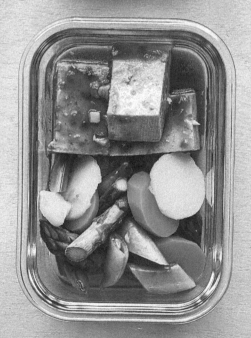

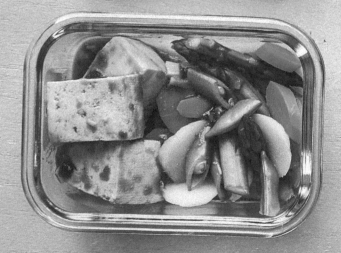

COLORFUL TOFU STIR-FRY **90**

CHAPTER FOUR

Meal Preps for General Diet

Congratulations! You have reached a milestone. It's time to celebrate the beginning of a new chapter with all the tools and new skills you've developed. The recipes in the following 3 preps are meant to ensure that you follow the bariatric guidelines of high-protein meals that are low in fat and carbs.

GENERAL DIET:
PREP 4

The theme of this week's prep is comfort foods. You can modify many of your favorite dishes to satisfy both your taste buds and your macros. This week, you'll prep four meals and one snack option, and you'll have meals for five days, instead of seven. For the remaining two days, I recommend using up frozen leftovers from earlier preps. Portions for meals will be about 3 ounces to 1 cup. It is essential that you listen to your fullness cues. These meals have a lower water content than those in the previous preps, which means they are more dense. Eat slowly, remember to chew 15 to 20 times before swallowing, and stop at the first sign of feeling full. For some, fullness means pressure, and for others it can be signaled by a hiccup, burp, sneeze, or a runny nose.

SHOPPING LIST

PRODUCE

- Apple (1)
- Eggplant, large (1)
- Garlic (1 head)
- Onions, small (2)
- Yellow squash, medium (1)
- Zucchini, large (1)

DAIRY AND DAIRY ALTERNATIVES

- Cheddar cheese, low-fat, sharp, shredded (8 ounces)
- Milk, reduced-fat (2%) (2 cups)
- Mozzarella cheese, fat-free (8 ounces)
- Oat milk (16 ounces)
- Sour cream, low-fat (4 ounces)

PROTEIN

- Chicken breasts, boneless, skinless, 3 to 4 (1 pound)
- Eggs (1)
- Ground beef, extra-lean (2 pounds)
- Ground chicken (1 pound)
- Protein powder, chocolate (2 scoops)
- Protein powder, unflavored (1 scoop)

PANTRY/CANNED/BOTTLED

- Beans, low-sodium, kidney, pinto, or white [2 (15-ounce) cans]
- Bread crumbs, regular or panko
- Chicken stock or broth (32 ounces)
- Chili powder
- Cinnamon, ground
- Cocoa powder
- Cumin, ground
- Diced tomatoes [1 (14.5-ounce) can]
- Marinara sauce (24 ounces)
- Nonstick cooking spray
- Oats, old-fashioned rolled
- Olive oil
- Oregano, dried
- Parsley, dried
- Peanut butter, creamy
- Peanut butter powder
- Salsa, mild (15 ounces)
- Salt
- Vanilla extract

EQUIPMENT

- Baking sheets (2)
- Blender/food processor
- Casserole dish
- Freezer-safe storage bags
- Ice cream scoop
- Mixing bowls, large (2)
- Paper towels
- Parchment paper
- Plastic wrap
- Saucepan (2½-quart)
- Sauté pan or skillet, large
- Slow cooker
- Storage containers: 16 medium and 16 small

	BREAKFAST	LUNCH	DINNER	SNACK/DESSERT	WATER
DAY 1	Chocolate Peanut Butter Shake	Chicken and Cheddar Chili	Saucy Chicken Meatballs	Overnight Oats	64 ounces
DAY 2	Chocolate Peanut Butter Shake	Chicken and Cheddar Chili	Low-Carb Meat Meatballs	Overnight Oats	64 ounces
DAY 3	Overnight Oats	Saucy Chicken Meatballs	Chicken and Cheddar Chili	Low-Carb Meat Lasagna	64 ounces
DAY 4	Overnight Oats	Low-Carb Meat Lasagna	Chicken and Cheddar Chili	Chocolate Peanut Butter Shake	64 ounces
DAY 5	Chocolate Peanut Butter Shake	Low-Carb Meat Lasagna	Chicken and Cheddar Chili	Saucy Chicken Meatballs	64 ounces

Step-by-Step Prep

1. Complete steps 1 and 2 of the Chicken and Cheddar Chili recipe (page 59).

2. Cut up vegetables, steps 1 to 2, for the Low-Carb Meat Lasagna (page 61).

3. Make the Saucy Chicken Meatballs (page 63) in their entirety.

4. Make the Overnight Oats (page 65).

5. Return to the Low-Carb Meat Lasagna, steps 3 through 7.

6. Divide the Saucy Chicken Meatballs among containers and store.

7. Make the Chocolate Peanut Butter Shake (page 66) to completion.

8. When the lasagna has cooled, divide and store.

9. Let the finished Chicken and Cheddar Chili cool in the refrigerator overnight; divide and store.

Chicken and Cheddar Chili

PREP TIME: 20 minutes / **COOK TIME:** 3 to 6 hours

MAKES 8 SERVINGS / GLUTEN-FREE, NUT-FREE, ONE POT

We tend to think of chili when it's cold, but this rich, comforting, and hearty version should be enjoyed year-round. Feel free to adjust the ingredients to your taste preferences. The only required ingredient is chili powder. I also include some added seasonings like salt, garlic powder, and cumin. Because spice can trigger discomfort, I left those, like cayenne, out of this version. Over time you can add some if you want to give it a little more heat.

3 to 4 boneless, skinless chicken breasts (about 1 pound)

3 cups chicken stock or Bone Broth (page 29)

2 (15-ounce) cans low-sodium beans (such as kidney, pinto, or white beans)

1 (15-ounce) jar mild salsa

1 (14.5-ounce) can diced tomatoes, undrained

1 small onion, chopped

3 tablespoons chili powder

2 tablespoons olive oil

1 tablespoon dried oregano

1 teaspoon ground cumin

2 cups shredded low-fat sharp cheddar cheese

½ cup low-fat sour cream

1. In a slow cooker, combine the chicken, chicken stock, beans, salsa, tomatoes and their juices, onion, chili powder, oil, oregano, and cumin. Stir well.

2. Cover and cook on low for 6 to 7 hours or on high for 3 hours. The internal temperature of the chicken should be 165°F, and the meat should break apart easily with a fork. Let cool.

3. Portion the chili evenly among 8 airtight containers and seal. Portion ¼ cup of cheese and 1 tablespoon of sour cream among 8 small separate airtight containers and seal.

4. Refrigerate for up to 4 days or freeze for up to 2 months.

continued

5. To serve, reheat the chili on the stovetop until warm, and top with 1 ounce of cheese and 1 to 2 tablespoons of sour cream.

VARIATION: This recipe can be made with ground beef as well. Brown the meat first, and drain the fat before adding the meat to the slow cooker.

PER SERVING: Calories: 334; Total fat: 14g; Total carbs: 25g; Sugar: 5g; Protein: 29g; Fiber: 8g; Sodium: 652mg

Low-Carb Meat Lasagna

PREP TIME: 30 minutes / **COOK TIME:** 1 hour, 20 minutes
MAKES 8 SERVINGS / GLUTEN-FREE, NUT-FREE

*Growing up in an Italian household, I remember enjoying homemade lasagna
at all the holiday meals, including Thanksgiving. Creating a gluten-free option
to carry on the tradition was important to me, because my children were gluten
intolerant. The fact that the noodles are replaced by vegetables was an added
bonus for this mom dietitian. And that's also a bonus after bariatric surgery,
because the finished dish is low in carbs and fat and high in protein and fiber.*

1 large zucchini

1 medium eggplant

1 large yellow squash

Salt

Nonstick cooking spray

½ large white onion, chopped

2 teaspoons minced garlic

2 pounds extra-lean ground beef

1 (24-ounce) jar marinara sauce

1½ cups shredded fat-free mozzarella cheese

1. Preheat the oven to 350°F. Position a rack in the middle of the oven.

2. Carefully slice the zucchini, eggplant, and yellow squash lengthwise into
   thick strips, about ¼ inch thick. Place the slices in a bowl and salt them
   generously, tossing once or twice to coat well. Lay the strips on paper towels
   and set them aside for 1 hour. Removing some liquid prevents this dish from
   becoming watery.

3. Spray a large saucepan with cooking spray and set it over medium heat. Add
   the onion; cook, stirring often, until softened, about 2 minutes. Add the garlic
   and cook for 20 seconds, until fragrant.

4. Add the ground beef, breaking it apart as it browns, and cook for 3 to
   4 minutes, until the meat is nearly cooked through.

5. Stir in the marinara sauce. Cook, stirring occasionally, for 10 minutes.

continued

6. Blot any moisture off the veggie strips with paper towels. Use the strips to line the bottom of a 9-by-13-inch baking pan, laying them just like you would lasagna noodles. Add a layer of meat sauce and cheese. Repeat these layers until you use all vegetables, sauce, and cheese.

7. Transfer the baking pan to the middle rack of the oven. Bake until bubbling, about 45 minutes.

8. Remove the lasagna from the oven and let it stand at room temperature for 10 minutes. Slice the lasagna into 8 servings; place 1 serving in each of 8 airtight containers.

9. Refrigerate 2 containers for up to 4 days, and freeze 6 containers for up to 3 months. Reheat from the refrigerator in the microwave for 2 to 3 minutes, or reheat directly from frozen in a 350°F oven for 20 to 25 minutes.

VARIATION: You can add a thin layer of low-fat ricotta cheese and extra vegetables, like spinach or mushrooms.

PER SERVING: Calories: 235; Total fat: 6g; Total carbs: 13g; Sugar: 8g; Protein: 34g; Fiber: 5g; Sodium: 269mg

Saucy Chicken Meatballs

PREP TIME: 45 minutes / **COOK TIME:** 10 minutes

MAKES 6 SERVINGS / DAIRY-FREE, NUT-FREE

Purchasing ground chicken and turkey can be tricky. You want to find the leanest option, but the labels are misleading. You will see lean or 93 percent on the front of the package, but you will also see extra lean or 97 percent. The simplest way to find the leaner option is to check the nutrition labels and choose the one that has less than 8 grams of fat per 4-ounce serving.

3 tablespoons olive oil, divided

½ medium onion, diced

1 large zucchini, grated

1 teaspoon minced garlic

1 (23.5-ounce) jar no-sugar-added
  marinara sauce

4 teaspoons dried parsley, divided

1 pound ground chicken

¼ cup plain or panko bread crumbs

1 large egg, beaten well

Nonstick cooking spray

1. Preheat the oven to 350°F

2. In a saucepan, heat 1 tablespoon of oil over medium heat. Cook the onion for about 3 minutes, until you see a translucent color and slight browning. Add the zucchini and cook for about 2 minutes, until it's soft.

3. Transfer the zucchini and onion to a bowl to cool while you start the sauce.

4. Add the remaining 2 tablespoons of oil and garlic to the saucepan. Cook for 1 minute, then add the marinara sauce and 2 teaspoons of parsley flakes; bring to a boil.

5. Simmer the sauce, uncovered, for about 30 minutes, stirring frequently.

6. To the bowl with the cooled zucchini and onion, add the ground chicken, bread crumbs, egg, and the remaining 2 tablespoons of parsley. Mix well.

continued

7. Lightly coat a baking sheet with cooking spray. Using an ice cream scoop or your hands, form the meatballs by rolling the mixture into 2-inch-diameter balls. Space the meatballs an inch or so apart, and bake for about 25 minutes or until they register 165°F on an instant-read thermometer.

8. Portion 2 meatballs into each of 6 airtight containers or storage bags, and cover each serving with about ½ cup of sauce.

9. Refrigerate 4 containers for up to 4 days, and freeze 2 containers for up to 3 months. Heat in the microwave, covered, for 1 to 1½ minutes. If reheating from frozen, first let it thaw overnight in the refrigerator.

PREP TIP: Keep a small bowl of water nearby when you are forming the balls. Wet your hands to prevent sticking.

PER SERVING: Calories: 229; Total fat: 14g; Total carbs: 10g; Sugar: 6g; Protein: 17g; Fiber: 3g; Sodium: 91mg

Overnight Oats

PREP TIME: 30 minutes

MAKES 4 SERVINGS / DAIRY-FREE, GLUTEN-FREE

This recipe can be modified in a number of ways—the combinations are endless. Swap out the apple for any preferred fruit options, like peeled pears, fresh berries, or melon, depending on what's in season. If you're feeling adventurous, try adding ¼ cup of shredded carrots or zucchini. The peanut butter powder can also be swapped for flaxseed meal, hemp seeds, or chia seeds (when you're cleared); you may need to add a little more liquid, though, because the seeds are very absorbent.

1 cup old-fashioned rolled oats

1 scoop unflavored protein powder
  (20 grams of protein)

2 teaspoons peanut butter powder

½ teaspoon ground cinnamon

1 small apple, peeled and finely chopped

2 cups oat milk or nondairy milk
  of choice

½ teaspoon vanilla extract

1. In a large bowl, combine the oats, protein powder, peanut butter powder, and cinnamon; mix well.

2. Portion ¼ cup of the mixed dry ingredients among 4 small airtight containers.

3. Layer the apples on top of the oats.

4. In a small bowl, mix the oat milk and vanilla together, then add ½ cup of the mixture to each container of oats and apples.

5. Refrigerate for up to 4 days. Enjoy cold, or heat for 30 seconds in the microwave.

INGREDIENT TIP: During the first month or two after surgery, you may need to use instant oats, because they are more compatible with a soft diet. However, as your digestion improves, transition to old-fashioned oats, which take longer to digest.

PER SERVING: Calories: 168; Total fat: 5g; Total carbs: 21g; Sugar: 4g; Protein: 11g; Fiber: 4g; Sodium: 57mg

Chocolate Peanut Butter Shake

PREP TIME: 5 minutes

MAKES 4 SERVINGS / 5-INGREDIENT, GLUTEN-FREE, UNDER 10

This shake is perfect when the desire for a frozen dessert kicks in. It's also a great batch to double up and freeze. The recipe calls for cocoa powder in addition to the chocolate protein. I recommend the special dark kind, which adds some richness to the recipe and counters the strong flavor of peanut butter. You can swap out the peanut butter for powdered peanut butter to reduce the calorie and fat content, or you can add some extra, like with the cocoa powder, to create a more intense flavor. You can also replace the ice cubes with frozen banana chunks or frozen strawberries to increase the sweetness.

2 cups reduced-fat milk

2 scoops chocolate protein powder
  (40 grams of protein)

2 tablespoons creamy peanut butter

1 tablespoon unsweetened
  cocoa powder

4 cups ice cubes

1. Combine the milk, protein powder, peanut butter, cocoa powder, and ice cubes in a blender, adjusting the cocoa and peanut butter powder to your taste preference. Blend until smooth.

2. Portion 1 cup of the shake into each of 4 glass jars and seal.

3. Refrigerate for up to 2 days or freeze for up to 1 week. If frozen, thaw in the refrigerator the night before serving. Place a shaker ball in the container to mix up the shake as it defrosts.

INGREDIENT TIP: Replace the milk with a nondairy option, like oat or almond milk, for a dairy-free alternative.

PER SERVING (1 CUP): Calories: 146; Total fat: 7g; Total carbs: 9g; Sugar: 7g; Protein: 14g; Fiber: 1g; Sodium: 89mg

GENERAL DIET: PREP 5

The recipes in this prep were designed with heart health in mind, meaning lower saturated fat and sodium and increased fiber. According to the CDC, heart disease is the leading cause of death in the United States. This week, you'll increase the recipes to five, with one snack option and complete meals for five days. Portions for meals will range from about 3 ounces to 1 cup. Aim for about 20 grams of protein with each meal. Remember to sip enough water throughout the day, because your meals don't have a high water content compared to earlier stages.

SHOPPING LIST

PRODUCE

- Bananas, ripe (2)
- Bell pepper, red, large (1)
- Garlic (1 head)
- Lemons (4)
- Mushrooms, sliced (8 ounces)
- Onion, small (1)
- Parsley, 1 bunch (freeze extra in water as ice cubes)
- Scallions (½ cup)
- Spinach, baby (8 ounces)

DAIRY AND DAIRY ALTERNATIVES

- Cheddar cheese, reduced-fat, shredded, sharp (4 ounces)
- Coconut milk, boxed, not canned (8 ounces)
- Cream cheese, fat-free (6 ounces)

PROTEIN

- Chicken thighs, boneless, skinless (2 pounds)
- Protein powder, plain (3 scoops)
- Salmon fillets, fresh (1 pound)

FROZEN

- Riced cauliflower, 1 (16-ounce) bag
- Tropical fruit blend (1 cup)

PANTRY/CANNED/BOTTLED

- Black beans, low-sodium (1 [14.5-ounce] can)
- Black pepper, cracked
- Cashews
- Chia seeds
- Chicken broth or Bone Broth (page 29) (32 ounces)
- Cinnamon, ground
- Flour, all-purpose
- Garlic powder
- Ginger, ground
- Honey
- Italian seasoning
- Kalamata olives or black olives, pitted
- Low-calorie sweetener
- Nonstick cooking spray
- Nutritional yeast (optional)
- Oats, old-fashioned rolled
- Olive oil, extra-virgin
- Onion powder
- Paprika
- Parmesan cheese, grated (optional)
- Peanut or almond butter
- Quinoa (1 cup)
- Salt
- Tomatoes, crushed (1 [15-ounce] can)
- Vegetable broth, low sodium (or bouillon) (32 ounces)

EQUIPMENT

- Aluminum foil
- Baking sheet
- Casserole dish, small
- Chef's knife
- Ice cream scoop
- Mixing bowls: large (2), medium (1), and small (1)
- Parchment paper
- Saucepan, (2½ quart and 1 quart)
- Sauté pan or skillet, large
- Slow cooker
- Storage bags
- Storage containers: 12 medium

	BREAKFAST	LUNCH	DINNER	SNACK/DESSERT	WATER
DAY 1	Tropical Breakfast Bowl	Creamy Chicken and Cauliflower Rice	Zesty Lemon Salmon Packet	Banana-Oat Protein Balls	64 ounces
DAY 2	Tropical Breakfast Bowl	Slow Cooker Chicken Cacciatore	Zesty Lemon Salmon Packet	Banana-Oat Protein Balls	64 ounces
DAY 3	Tropical Breakfast Bowl	Slow Cooker Chicken Cacciatore	Zesty Lemon Salmon Packet	Quinoa and Black Bean Bowls	64 ounces
DAY 4	Banana-Oat Protein Balls	Zesty Lemon Salmon Packet	Creamy Chicken and Cauliflower Rice	Quinoa and Black Bean Bowls	64 ounces
DAY 5	Banana-Oat Protein Balls	Slow Cooker Chicken Cacciatore	Creamy Chicken and Cauliflower Rice	Quinoa and Black Bean Bowls	64 ounces

Step-by-Step Prep

1. Complete steps 1 through 6 of the Slow Cooker Chicken Cacciatore (page 70).

2. Complete step 1 for both the Quinoa and Black Bean Bowl (page 74) and Tropical Breakfast Bowl (page 79).

3. Complete steps 1 through 3 of the Creamy Chicken and Cauliflower Rice (page 72).

4. Make the Banana-Oat Protein Balls (page 76) to completion.

5. Complete steps 4 through 7 of the Creamy Chicken and Cauliflower Rice.

6. Complete steps 2 through 5 of the Quinoa and Black Bean Bowl.

7. Finish and store the Tropical Breakfast Bowl and the Quinoa and Black Bean Bowls.

8. Make the Zesty Lemon Salmon Packet (page 77) to completion.

9. Finish and store the Creamy Chicken and Cauliflower Rice. Store the cooled Slow Cooker Chicken Cacciatore.

Slow Cooker Chicken Cacciatore

PREP TIME: 20 minutes / **COOK TIME:** 6 hours
MAKES 4 SERVINGS / NUT-FREE

This dish is traditionally cooked with wine; however, store-bought stock or homemade Bone Broth (page 29) are great substitutes. Although it's delicious on its own, try pairing the chicken with zucchini noodles, spaghetti squash, or riced vegetables. You can also add more vegetables to your slow cooker, like peppers and carrots, which will enhance sweetness. Although it's an option, I wouldn't skip browning the chicken—it adds a ton of flavor.

¼ cup all-purpose flour

4 boneless, skinless chicken thighs
  (1 pound)

2 tablespoons olive oil

1 small onion, thinly sliced

½ cup low-sodium chicken broth or Bone
  Broth (page 29)

1 (15-ounce) can crushed tomatoes

8 ounces mushrooms, sliced

¼ cup pitted kalamata or black olives,
  drained and chopped

1 tablespoon Italian seasoning

2 garlic cloves, minced

2 tablespoons grated Parmesan cheese,
  for garnish

2 tablespoons chopped fresh parsley,
  for garnish

1. Place the flour in a resealable bag. Add the chicken thighs and toss to coat.

2. In a large skillet, heat the oil over medium-high heat. Brown the chicken for 3 minutes per side. Transfer the chicken to the slow cooker.

3. Add the onion to the skillet and cook for 2 to 3 minutes, until it begins to brown. Scrape the cooked onion into the slow cooker.

4. Add the broth to the skillet, scrape up any brown bits to release the flavors, and then pour the broth into the slow cooker, along with the tomatoes, mushrooms, olives, Italian seasoning, and garlic. Stir to combine.

5. Cover and cook on low for 5 to 6 hours, until the chicken thighs register 165°F on an instant-read thermometer.

6. Portion the chicken evenly among 4 storage containers, cool, and seal.

7. Refrigerate for up to 4 days or freeze for up to 3 months. Reheat on the stove-top over low heat, covered with some sauce.

8. To serve, garnish with cheese and parsley.

INGREDIENT TIP: You can use chicken quarters here, because cooking bone-in chicken will add more depth to the dish. However, you should remove the skin prior to slow cooking, because it will get soggy and add fat to the dish.

PER SERVING: Calories: 301; Total fat: 13g; Total carbs: 19g; Sugar: 7g; Protein: 28g; Fiber: 3g; Sodium: 378mg

Creamy Chicken and Cauliflower Rice

PREP TIME: 15 minutes / **COOK TIME:** 45 minutes
MAKES 4 SERVINGS / GLUTEN-FREE, NUT-FREE

The words creamy *and* casserole *may have you wondering, "How can this be heart-healthy?" Replacing heavy cream with fat-free cream cheese drastically reduces the amount of saturated fat in this recipe. In addition, including cauliflower rice adds fiber to your meal. Don't limit yourself to the cauliflower rice in this recipe, either. As you advance and can increase portions per meal, feel free to toss in an additional cup of colorful frozen vegetables from your freezer. You can swap out the chicken thighs for breasts, too.*

Nonstick cooking spray

4 boneless, skinless chicken thighs
  (1 pound)

Extra-virgin olive oil

1 (16-ounce) bag riced cauliflower

6 ounces fat-free cream cheese, at room
  temperature

½ cup thinly sliced scallions, divided

2 tablespoons chopped fresh parsley

½ teaspoon Italian seasoning

1 cup shredded reduced-fat sharp
  cheddar cheese, divided

1. Preheat the oven to 450°F and spray a casserole dish with cooking spray.

2. Lay out the chicken in the prepared dish, brush it with oil, and cook for 15 to 18 minutes. Don't overcook; the internal temperature of the chicken should be 165°F. Set aside to cool.

3. In a large skillet, sauté the riced cauliflower over medium heat for about 15 minutes. (You can also heat the cauliflower rice in the microwave for 5 minutes to save time.)

4. In a food processor, combine the cream cheese, ¼ cup of scallions, the parsley, and the Italian seasoning. Pulse until smooth, then scoop the mixture into a large bowl.

5. Cube the cooled chicken and add it to the cream cheese mixture, along with the riced cauliflower and ½ cup of cheddar. Mix well.

6. Spoon the mixture into the prepared casserole dish. Sprinkle with the remaining ½ cup of cheddar and cover with foil.

7. Lower the oven temperature to 400°F and bake for 30 minutes.

8. Let cool thoroughly in the refrigerator before dividing and storing.

9. Portion 1 cup of the casserole into each of 4 airtight storage containers and seal.

10. Refrigerate for up to 4 days or freeze up to 3 months. Reheat from frozen for 4 to 6 minutes on high in the microwave. Use a vented lid, and stir midway. To reheat the casserole on the stovetop, transfer it to a saucepan and heat for 15 minutes, uncovered, over low heat. You can add a few tablespoons of water for more moisture.

VARIATION: This dish is nice with a little heat. When you are cleared for spicy foods, and if you are not experiencing reflux, add ¼ teaspoon of cayenne pepper along with the other spices.

PER SERVING (1 CUP): Calories: 303; Total fat: 11g; Total carbs: 11g; Sugar: 5g; Protein: 39g; Fiber: 3g; Sodium: 621mg

Quinoa and Black Bean Bowl

PREP TIME: 10 minutes / **COOK TIME:** 30 minutes

MAKES 4 SERVINGS / GLUTEN-FREE, NUT-FREE, VEGAN

I first discovered quinoa when I was working as a retail dietitian for a large chain grocery store. The first lesson provided by the company was its pronunciation: keen-wah. The second lesson was on the protein content of this quick-cooking seed. Quinoa is a complete protein, meaning that it contains all nine essential amino acids, which is great for those wanting to include more plant-based protein options in their diets.

1 cup water

½ cup quinoa, rinsed

2 tablespoons olive oil

2 garlic cloves, minced

1 large red bell pepper, finely chopped

1 cup low-sodium vegetable broth

1 cup chopped baby spinach

¾ cup canned black beans, drained and rinsed

1 teaspoon onion powder

Salt

Freshly ground black pepper

Nutritional yeast or grated Parmesan cheese (optional)

1. In a small saucepan, bring the water and quinoa to a boil over high heat. Cover, reduce the heat to low, and simmer until the water is absorbed, about 15 minutes.

2. In a large saucepan, heat the oil over medium heat. Add the garlic and sauté for 30 seconds.

3. Add the bell pepper and cook, stirring occasionally, for 5 to 7 minutes, until tender.

4. Add the broth, spinach, beans, onion powder, salt, and pepper to the saucepan. Cook for another 3 minutes.

5. Turn off the heat and add the cooked quinoa. Fluff with a fork to mix. Let cool.

6. Portion ½ to ¾ cup into each of 4 airtight containers and seal.

7. Refrigerate for up to 1 week or freeze for up to 6 months. Enjoy cold or heat in a microwave for 30 seconds. To reheat from frozen, first thaw in the refrigerator overnight.

8. To serve, sprinkle with nutritional yeast (if using) and enjoy.

VARIATION: If you are unable to eat spinach and bell peppers, replace them with cooked broccoli florets and marinated red peppers.

PER SERVING (½ CUP): Calories: 199; Total fat: 8g; Total carbs: 25g; Sugar: 2g; Protein: 7g; Fiber: 5g; Sodium: 49mg

Banana-Oat Protein Balls

PREP TIME: 30 minutes

MAKES 16 BALLS / GLUTEN-FREE

Looking to satisfy your sweet tooth and fuel up? Look no further. These are not low calorie, so be mindful of serving sizes as you are able to consume larger portions. You can use these in place of store-bought protein bars. If you're feeling adventurous, add some coconut flakes, chopped nuts, sugar-free chocolate chips, or vanilla.

¼ cup chia seeds

¼ cup water or unsweetened
  almond milk

2 ripe bananas, mashed

½ cup creamy or chunky peanut butter or
  almond butter

1 tablespoon honey

1 cup old-fashioned rolled oats

1 scoop unflavored protein powder
  (20 grams of protein)

1 teaspoon ground cinnamon

1. In a medium bowl, mix together the chia seeds and water. Add the bananas, peanut butter, and honey; mix well.

2. In another medium bowl, mix together the oats, protein powder, and cinnamon. Fold the dry ingredients into the wet ingredients. Cover with plastic wrap and place the bowl in the refrigerator for 1 hour to chill.

3. Using an ice cream scoop, scoop out 2 tablespoons of dough and form it into a ball. (Like with meatballs, wet hands will help you roll the balls with less peanut butter sticking.) Repeat with the remaining dough.

4. Portion 2 protein balls into each of 8 resealable bags.

5. Refrigerate for up to 1 week, or flash-freeze the balls on a baking sheet for 1 to 2 hours, then transfer them to a freezer bag and store them in the freezer for up to 3 months. Thaw in the refrigerator before enjoying.

VARIATION: For a nut-free option, replace the nut butter with sunflower butter or chickpea butter.

PER SERVING: Calories: 107; Total fat: 6g; Total carbs: 11g; Sugar: 3g; Protein: 4g; Fiber: 3g; Sodium: 4mg

Zesty Lemon Salmon Packets

PREP TIME: 5 minutes / **COOK TIME:** 14 minutes
MAKES 4 SERVINGS / DAIRY-FREE, GLUTEN-FREE, NUT-FREE

Lemon creates a fresh and zesty flavor. The tartness has also been known to help with nausea, which can still occur on occasion after surgery. Whether you make this with salmon, tilapia, cod, halibut, or swordfish, you'll enjoy this simple, fast, and refreshing dish. Fish is often well tolerated among those who have had bariatric surgery, because it is easier to digest than most solid proteins. It's also low in saturated fat, making it heart-healthy. However, it can dry out fast, so keep your cooking temperatures low and cover your fish when reheating. You can even add some additional olive oil, lemon, and fresh herbs, if desired.

2 tablespoons olive oil, divided

1 teaspoon lemon juice, divided

4 (4-ounce) salmon fillets

2 teaspoons garlic powder

2 teaspoons paprika

1 teaspoon freshly ground black pepper

2 lemons, thinly sliced

1. Preheat the oven to 400°F.

2. In a large bowl, drizzle half of the oil and lemon juice over the salmon, reserving a little bit of each for later. Season with the garlic powder, paprika, and pepper.

3. Rip off 4 squares of aluminum foil. Place 1 or 2 lemon slices on each piece of foil, then place the salmon fillets on top and fold up the sides of the foil. Drizzle the reserved lemon juice and oil over the salmon, then top with more lemon slices and seal the foil packets.

4. Place the packets on a baking sheet and transfer them to the oven. Bake for 10 to 12 minutes, until the internal temperature of the salmon reaches 145°F. The salmon will flake easily with a fork and turn light pink. Remove from the oven and let cool.

continued

5. Portion 1 fillet into each of 4 airtight containers, let cool, and seal.

6. Refrigerate for up to 3 days or freeze for up to 2 months. Reheat in the oven at 275°F for about 10 minutes.

VARIATION: When you are cleared to eat leafy greens, try this zesty salmon cold over lettuce.

PER SERVING (3 OUNCES): Calories: 230; Total fat: 14g; Total carbs: 2g; Sugar: 0g; Protein: 23g; Fiber: 1g; Sodium: 52mg

Tropical Breakfast Bowl

PREP TIME: 5 minutes / **COOK TIME:** 15 minutes
MAKES 4 SERVINGS / VEGETARIAN

Breakfast after weight loss surgery shouldn't be limited to eggs and oatmeal. Quinoa is a good source of protein and heart-healthy fiber. This recipe is mild in flavor, because your taste buds may be hypersensitive after surgery. If you are not a fan of the tropical fruits, swap them out for any preferred frozen fruit, like mango, peaches, or strawberries. I would avoid frozen blueberries, though, because they will turn your dish a dark gray color.

½ cup quinoa, rinsed

1 cup water

¾ cup coconut milk (boxed, not canned) or dairy-free milk of your choice

½ teaspoon ground ginger

¼ teaspoon low-calorie sweetener (optional)

1 cup frozen tropical fruit blend, chopped into ¼-inch pieces

4 scoops unflavored protein powder (80 grams of protein)

½ cup chopped cashews or macadamia nuts

1. In a small saucepan, bring the quinoa and water to a boil over high heat. Cover, reduce the heat to low, and simmer until the water is absorbed, about 15 minutes.

2. Portion 1½ cups of quinoa into each of 4 airtight containers.

3. In a small bowl, whisk together the coconut milk, ginger, and sweetener (if using). Pour this mixture evenly over the quinoa. Add the fruit and mix well.

4. Add 1 scoop of protein powder to each serving; mix well.

5. Refrigerate for up to 4 days or freeze for up to 6 months. If frozen, let it thaw in the refrigerator overnight.

continued

6. To serve, top with 1 tablespoon of nuts prior to enjoying.

PREP TIP: You can double the quantity of quinoa you make in this recipe. Cook 1 cup of quinoa in 2 cups of water; this will yield about 3 cups of cooked quinoa. You can use the remaining 1½ cups for the Quinoa and Black Bean Bowl (page 74) in this prep.

PER SERVING (½ CUP): Calories: 339; Total fat: 23g; Total carbs: 26g; Sugar: 5g; Protein: 11g; Fiber: 4g; Sodium: 45mg

GENERAL DIET:
PREP 6

By the time you reach this prep, you should be cleared for all foods and textures, usually around three months after surgery. You'll need to continue to focus on protein, though, and your intake per meal will begin to increase, so in this prep I emphasize lean proteins.

Over time, you will wait longer stretches between meals. Eating six times per day will no longer be necessary. Having three meals with 25 to 30 grams of protein and one snack with 10 to 15 grams of protein is a good long-term pattern to consider. Including more solid proteins and vegetables that take time to chew and digest helps regulate calories as well. Keep in mind, it's easier to consume more liquids and soft foods in one sitting, especially if they are processed foods often known as "slider foods." You will be able to consume even more if you drink with your meal, which is why I suggest you continue to drink your water between meals, at least 64 ounces a day.

SHOPPING LIST

PRODUCE

- Asparagus, small bunch (1)
- Bell pepper, medium, any color (1)
- Carrots, large (2)
- Dill paste (or fresh dill, 1 bunch)
- Garlic (1 bulb)
- Ginger paste (or fresh ginger, ¼ teaspoon)
- Lemon (1)
- Lettuce, butter or romaine (1 head)
- Limes (2)
- Mushrooms, sliced (8 ounces)
- Onion, small (1)
- Snap peas (8 ounces, or green beans)
- Tomatoes, small (7)
- Zucchini, medium (4)

DAIRY

- Cottage cheese, low-fat (32 ounces)
- Greek yogurt, plain, low-fat (5 ounces)
- Mozzarella, part-skim (4 ounces)
- Pepper Jack cheese (4 ounces)
- Sour cream, low-fat (6 ounces)

PROTEIN

- Ground beef, lean (1 pound)
- Ground chicken (or turkey), extra lean (1 pound)
- Eggs (6)
- Protein powder, unflavored (1 scoop)
- Salmon, smoked (6 ounces)
- Tofu, extra-firm, (2 [12- to 15-ounce] packages)

FROZEN

- Shrimp, peeled and deveined (1 pound)
- Strawberries (16 ounces)

PANTRY/CANNED/BOTTLED

- Beans, cannellini (white kidney beans) or navy beans (15 ounces)
- Cajun seasoning
- Cornstarch
- Farro (16 ounces)
- Guacamole (4 [2-ounce] portions)
- Honey
- Honey mustard dressing,
- low-calorie, yogurt-based (¼ cup)
- Marinara sauce (½ cup)
- Mayonnaise, light
- Mustard, powdered
- Nonstick cooking spray
- Olive oil, extra-virgin
- Salsa (1 [15-ounce] jar)
- Salt
- Sesame oil
- Soy sauce, light
- Tortillas, low carb, 80 calories or less (4)
- Water chestnuts, sliced (8 ounces)

EQUIPMENT

- Baking pan
- Baking sheet
- Mixing bowls: 2 large, 1 medium, 1 small
- Paper towels
- Parchment paper
- Saucepans: 2½ quart, 1 quart
- Sauté pan or skillet, large
- Storage bags, freezer-safe
- Storage containers: 24 medium, 8 dual-compartment

	BREAKFAST	LUNCH	DINNER	SNACK/ DESSERT	WATER
DAY 1	Farro and Fruit Breakfast Bowl	Cajun Chicken Sliders	Lettuce-Wrap Shrimp Tacos with Chips and Guacamole	Egg and Salmon Snacks	64 to 72 ounces
DAY 2	Farro and Fruit Breakfast Bowl	Cajun Chicken Sliders	Lettuce-Wrap Shrimp Tacos with Chips and Guacamole	Egg and Salmon Snacks	64 to 72 ounces
DAY 3	Farro and Fruit Breakfast Bowl	Zucchini Boats with Meat Sauce	Lettuce-Wrap Shrimp Tacos with Chips and Guacamole	Colorful Tofu Stir-Fry	64 to 72 ounces
DAY 4	Farro and Fruit Breakfast Bowl	Zucchini Boats with Meat Sauce	Colorful Tofu Stir-Fry	Cajun Chicken Sliders	64 to 72 ounces
DAY 5	Egg and Salmon Snacks	Zucchini Boats with Meat Sauce	Colorful Tofu Stir-Fry	Cajun Chicken Sliders	64 to 72 ounces

Step-by-Step Prep

1. Follow steps 1 through 5 of the Zucchini Boats with Meat Sauce (page 84).

2. Follow steps 1 and 2 of the Farro and Fruit Breakfast Bowl (page 86).

3. Complete steps 1 through 4 of the Cajun Chicken Sliders (page 88).

4. Follow the Colorful Tofu Stir-Fry (page 90), steps 1 through 6.

5. Resume the Farro and Fruit Breakfast Bowl to completion. Follow steps 1 and 2 of the Egg and Salmon Snacks (page 92).

6. Return to the Colorful Tofu Stir-Fry and complete step 7. Finish and store the Cajun Chicken Sliders and the Egg and Salmon Snacks.

7. Finish and store the Zucchini Boats. Make the Lettuce-Wrap Shrimp Tacos with Chips and Guacamole (page 93) to completion.

Zucchini Boats with Meat Sauce

PREP TIME: 30 minutes / **COOK TIME:** 30 minutes
MAKES 8 SERVINGS / GLUTEN-FREE, NUT-FREE

This stuffed zucchini recipe is layered with flavor. The savory and sweet notes complement each other well, and the aroma is mouthwatering. Mixing the meat with vegetables decreases the fat content and adds some low-calorie bulk to the dish. This is a great technique for long-term weight management when you're able to eat larger volumes.

4 medium zucchini

2 tablespoons olive oil, divided

1 small onion, chopped

1 pound lean ground beef

½ cup chopped mushrooms (any kind)

½ bell pepper (any color), chopped

½ cup marinara sauce

1 cup shredded part-skim mozzarella, divided

1. Preheat the oven to 350°F.

2. Cut the ends off the zucchini, then cut each one in half lengthwise; scoop out the pulp, leaving ½-inch-deep shells. Finely chop up the pulp and set it aside.

3. Place the boats on a baking sheet and brush lightly with 1 tablespoon of oil. Bake, uncovered, until the zucchini is fork-tender, 25 to 30 minutes. Remove the zucchini from the oven.

4. In a skillet, heat the remaining 1 tablespoon of oil over medium heat. Cook the onion for 5 minutes, until translucent. Add the beef and cook until it's no longer pink, about 7 minutes, then drain off the fat.

5. Add the zucchini pulp, mushrooms, pepper, and marinara sauce to the skillet. Cook for 4 to 5 minutes, until soft. Remove from the heat.

6. Divide the mushroom-pepper mixture evenly among the zucchini boats, then let them cool. Top with cheese.

7. Portion 1 zucchini boat into each of 8 airtight containers.

8. Refrigerate for up to 4 days or freeze for up to 3 months. Reheat in the microwave from the refrigerator or freezer in 30-second intervals until heated through. Or, thaw in about 1 inch of water for 20 minutes, wrap loosely in foil, and bake in a 275°F oven for 20 minutes.

VARIATION: Turn this into a vegetarian dish by swapping out the ground beef for canned black beans.

PER SERVING: Calories: 164; Total fat: 9g; Total carbs: 5g; Sugar: 4g; Protein: 17g; Fiber: 1g; Sodium: 155mg

Farro and Fruit Breakfast Bowl

PREP TIME: 10 minutes / **COOK TIME:** 30 minutes
MAKES 4 SERVINGS / GLUTEN-FREE, NUT-FREE

For long-term weight loss success, I encourage you to think beyond rice and pasta. Farro, which is rich in magnesium, zinc, and B vitamins, is a lovely grain to consider. It can be used in place of quinoa or oats in almost any recipe in this book. It has a nutty flavor and a great texture, and it will give you that bite that is often missed after surgery. Because it's high in carbohydrates, you'll need to keep portions small. This slow-digesting breakfast will help you stay full until lunch.

½ cup farro, rinsed

1½ cups water

¼ teaspoon salt

8 ounces frozen fruit of choice (strawberries, peaches, or mango)

2 cups low-fat cottage cheese or yogurt

1 scoop vanilla or unflavored protein powder (20 grams of protein)

1. In a small saucepan, combine the farro with the water and salt over high heat. Bring to a boil, then reduce the heat to low and simmer for about 20 minutes or until the farro is tender.

2. Drain any excess liquid and spread out the farro on a baking sheet so it cools quickly; this will help it maintain its chewy texture.

3. Place ¼ cup farro and ¼ cup fruit on one side of each of 4 dual-compartment storage containers.

4. In a small bowl, mix together the cottage cheese and protein powder. Place ½ cup of this mixture into each of the 4 containers, next to the farro and fruit.

5. Refrigerate for up to 4 days. Do not freeze.

COOKING TIP: To enhance the sweetness of this dish, you can heat the farro and fruit in a microwave for 30 seconds before mixing in the cottage cheese.

INGREDIENT TIP: Spread leftover cooked farro on a baking sheet and flash-freeze it for 2 hours, then divide it into ¼-cup portions and freeze in individual airtight containers. Defrost in the refrigerator.

PER SERVING: Calories: 174; Total fat: 2g; Total carbs: 27g; Sugar: 11g; Protein: 13g; Fiber: 4g; Sodium: 243mg

Cajun Chicken Sliders

PREP TIME: 10 minutes, plus 30 minutes to cool / **COOK TIME:** 20 minutes

MAKES 4 SERVINGS / GLUTEN-FREE

If burgers were a staple in your pre-surgery diet, this bean-and-chicken combination will surprise you. It's actually a trick I learned when my children were little. Finding ways to increase the nutritional value of your meals by adjusting some old favorites is a helpful practice for long-term weight loss success. These white beans are so versatile, too, with a creamy texture and mild flavor.

1 cup canned white beans (navy beans or cannellini/white kidney)

1 pound extra-lean ground chicken or turkey

1 teaspoon Cajun seasoning

1 teaspoon mustard powder

6 large romaine lettuce leaves or butter lettuce leaves (if cleared to do so)

2 ounces sliced pepper jack cheese

¼ cup honey mustard dressing or low-calorie dressing of choice

4 small tomatoes, sliced

1. Preheat the oven to 400°F.

2. In a large bowl, mash the beans with a potato masher or large fork. Mix in the ground chicken, Cajun seasoning, and mustard.

3. Form the mixture into 4-ounce patties, place them on a baking sheet, and bake for 20 minutes or until their internal temperature reaches 165°F.

4. Once cooked, place the patties in the refrigerator to cool, uncovered, for about 30 minutes.

5. Place 1 slider in each of 4 airtight containers.

6. Refrigerate for up to 4 days. To freeze, wrap the patties in plastic wrap, then place them in airtight freezer bags and store in the freezer for up to 3 months. Reheat from the refrigerator in the microwave for about 2 minutes. From the freezer, thaw overnight or cook the patties in a lightly greased skillet over medium heat for 4 to 5 minutes per side.

7. To serve, place a patty on a lettuce leaf (if you're cleared for greens) and top with ½ slice of cheese, 1 tablespoon dressing, and tomato slices.

SUBSTITUTION: To reduce the heat, leave out the Cajun seasoning and use low-fat Muenster or Swiss cheese.

PER SERVING: Calories: 338; Total fat: 16g; Total carbs: 20g; Sugar: 6g; Protein: 30g; Fiber: 4g; Sodium: 291mg

Colorful Tofu Stir-Fry

PREP TIME: 30 minutes / **COOK TIME:** 10 minutes

MAKES 8 SERVINGS / DAIRY-FREE, NUT-FREE, VEGETARIAN

Looking for a colorful, crunchy meal that will help you forget you ever followed a pureed diet? Well, this is it. The main part of this prep is having your vegetables chopped in even pieces and ready to go. A quick blanch of some vegetables so they hold their texture after storage is all you need to do. I provided some stir-fry vegetable suggestions, but as always, you are not limited to those. Choose three vegetables of varying colors, toss, season, and serve with tofu, shrimp, or scallops.

6 cups water

¼ cup salt

2 large carrots, evenly sliced

1 bunch asparagus, trimmed and quartered

8 ounces snap peas or green beans, chopped

1 (8-ounce) can sliced water chestnuts, drained

⅓ cup light soy sauce

1 tablespoon cornstarch

1 teaspoon honey

¼ teaspoon ginger paste or grated fresh ginger

¼ cup sesame oil

24 ounces extra-firm tofu, pressed and cut into 1-inch cubes

1 teaspoon minced garlic

1. In a large pot, bring the water and salt to a boil over high heat.

2. Fill a large bowl with ice and water.

3. Place the carrots in the boiling water. Stir for 2 to 3 minutes, then use a slotted spoon to transfer the carrots to the ice water. Repeat with the asparagus, then the snap peas. Leave each vegetable in the ice bath for 2 to 3 minutes, then drain them on paper towels.

4. Once drained, transfer the blanched veggies to a large mixing bowl and add the water chestnuts.

5. In a separate bowl, combine the soy sauce, cornstarch, honey, and ginger. Mix until the cornstarch dissolves.

6. In a large sauté pan, heat the oil over medium heat. Add the tofu, soy sauce mixture, and garlic and toss for 1 to 2 minutes. Remove the pan from the heat and let the tofu cool.

7. Portion 3 ounces of the tofu mixture and ½ to ¾ cup of the vegetable mixture into each of 8 airtight containers; seal.

8. Refrigerate for up to 5 days or freeze for up to 3 months. Reheat from the refrigerator in the microwave for 1 to 1½ minutes. Reheat from the freezer on the stovetop in a sauté pan with oil; add 1 tablespoon of light soy sauce and 2 tablespoons of water and toss until heated thoroughly, about 5 minutes.

INGREDIENT TIP: Freezing will change the tofu's texture, but it will also allow it to absorb more of the liquid you are reheating it with.

PER SERVING: Calories: 204; Total fat: 12g; Total carbs: 16g; Sugar: 3g; Protein: 11g; Fiber: 2g; Sodium: 1275mg

Egg and Salmon Snacks

PREP TIME: 5 minutes, plus 15 minutes to rest / **COOK TIME:** 10 minutes
MAKES 4 SERVINGS / GLUTEN-FREE, NUT-FREE

Eggs are such a fabulous protein source that I want to keep them interesting for you. Here, I encourage you to bring back an old holiday favorite, the deviled egg; this variation includes smoked salmon. You can use any flavor combination you want, however. Make some Greek-style snacks with feta cheese and olives, or spicy Buffalo with ranch dressing and hot sauce.

6 large eggs

3 tablespoons low-fat plain Greek yogurt

3 tablespoons light mayonnaise

1 tablespoon dill paste or chopped
    fresh dill

1 teaspoon lemon juice

Salt

Freshly ground black pepper

6 ounces smoked salmon

1. In a large pot, cover the eggs with water and bring to a boil, then turn off the heat, cover the pot, and let sit for 15 minutes. Rinse them under cold water. Set aside.

2. In a medium bowl, combine the yogurt, mayonnaise, dill, lemon juice, salt, and pepper.

3. Peel and halve the eggs lengthwise. Remove the yolks and add them to the yogurt mixture. Mash with a fork to combine.

4. Fill the eggs with the yolk-yogurt mixture, then top each egg half with 1 ounce of salmon.

5. Portion 1½ eggs into each of 4 airtight storage containers and seal.

6. Refrigerate for up to 4 days. Enjoy cold.

INGREDIENT TIP: Hard-boil and peel extra eggs to mix into grain dishes like farro or quinoa bowls for added protein.

PER SERVING: Calories: 207; Total fat: 14g; Total carbs: 2g; Sugar: 1g; Protein: 18g; Fiber: 0g; Sodium: 529mg

Lettuce-Wrap Shrimp Tacos with Chips and Guacamole

PREP TIME: 10 minutes / **COOK TIME:** 10 minutes
MAKES 4 SERVINGS

From mild to spicy, these tacos will have your mouth popping with flavor. Unlike in most restaurant varieties, the fish here isn't fried. You won't be missing anything in the flavor department, though. The guacamole provides richness and heart-healthy fat. It is loaded with lean protein, too. If shrimp is still a challenge for you to digest, replace it with a flaky fish fillet (such as cod or tilapia) to better suit your needs.

1 pound frozen shrimp, peeled and
  deveined
2 tablespoons Cajun seasoning
Juice of 1 lime
4 low-carb tortillas, quartered
Nonstick cooking spray

4 large romaine lettuce leaves or butter
  lettuce leaves
⅓ cup salsa
3 tomatoes, chopped
4 (2-ounce) packages guacamole

1. Place a baking sheet on the top rack of your oven, about 6 inches from the broiler. Preheat the broiler.

2. Rinse the shrimp under cold water, then place them on a paper towel to dry. Sprinkle the shrimp with Cajun seasoning.

3. Remove the hot baking sheet from the oven. Spread out the shrimp on the baking sheet, return the baking sheet to the oven, and broil the shrimp for 5 minutes, until they turn pink and begin to curl. Transfer the broiled shrimp to a plate and add the lime juice.

4. Place the tortillas on the baking sheet and spray them with cooking spray. Broil for 5 minutes, until crispy.

5. Portion 4 tortilla quarters (1 tortilla) into each of 4 resealable bags. Portion 1 lettuce leaf into each of 4 resealable bags.

continued

Meal Preps for General Diet   93

6. Place 3 ounces of shrimp on one side of each of 4 dual-compartment storage containers. On the other side of the containers, place 1 to 2 tablespoons of salsa and tomatoes.

7. Refrigerate for up to 4 days. To reheat, warm the shrimp on the stovetop for 5 minutes or in a toaster oven at 300°F for 15 minutes.

8. To serve, place the shrimp in the lettuce leaf and top with salsa and tomatoes. Enjoy with a few crunchy tortilla chips and guacamole.

INGREDIENT TIP: Don't skip baking the tortillas, because unheated tortillas have a doughy texture and are difficult to digest.

PER SERVING: Calories: 305; Total fat: 12g; Total carbs: 29g; Sugar: 6g; Protein: 29g; Fiber: 5g; Sodium: 589mg

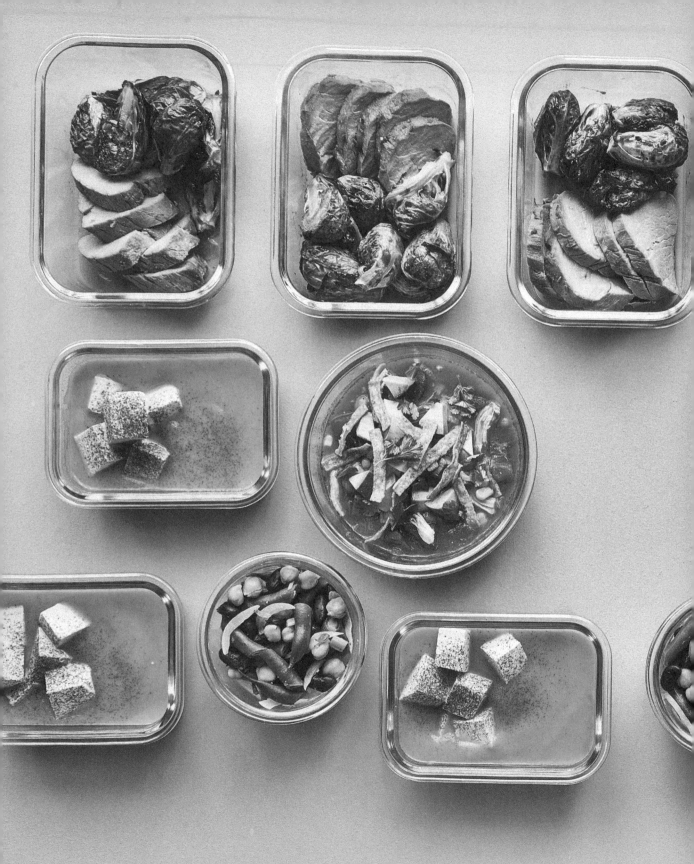

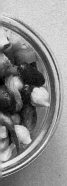

PART TWO

More Recipes to Prep

This section provides you with 35 additional recipes, some of which are suitable for the early stages after surgery. Feel free to swap these in for recipes in those earlier preps, or simply add one or two extra recipes to your prep days, because some of them can be made in under 10 minutes with simple ingredients you likely already have on hand.

Six months after your surgery, I encourage you to remember one important thing: Continuing to focus on protein does not mean you need to keep increasing the portion sizes. Use your ability to consume a larger volume to enjoy more nutrient-rich vegetables, fruits, and high-fiber carbohydrates. Having balance in your meals will help you stay healthy.

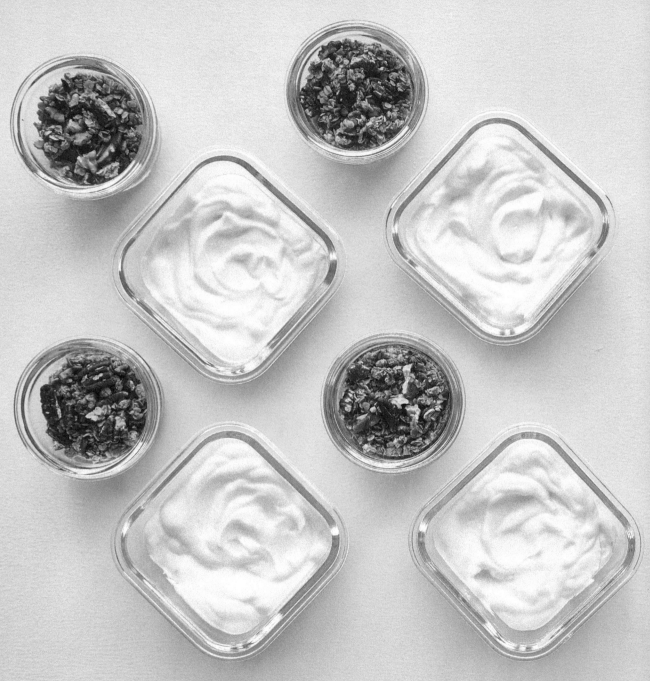

EASY HOMEMADE
GRANOLA **106**

CHAPTER FIVE

Shakes, Smoothies, and Breakfasts

TROPICAL PROTEIN POWER SMOOTHIE **100**

GREEN GOODNESS SMOOTHIE **101**

CHOCOLATE CHERRY SHAKE **102**

SWEET POTATO–ALMOND SMOOTHIE **103**

SAVORY GAZPACHO SHAKE **104**

CHIA PUDDING **105**

EASY HOMEMADE GRANOLA **106**

CRUSTLESS TOMATO, BROCCOLI, AND
MOZZARELLA QUICHE **108**

ZESTY FAVA BEANS **110**

LOW-CARB BREAKFAST BURRITOS **112**

Tropical Protein Power Smoothie

PREP TIME: 8 minutes

MAKES 6 SERVINGS / 5-INGREDIENT, GLUTEN-FREE, STAGE 1, UNDER 10, VEGETARIAN

Looking for a refreshing beverage that will remind you of a day by the beach? This sweet tropical fruit smoothie will hydrate and provide a great source of protein, too. Using coconut water provides added electrolytes like calcium, magnesium, and potassium, along with vitamin C from the fruit. The chia seeds add omega-3 fatty acids and fiber, which will help you feel fuller longer as well. If you don't have a tropical fruit mix, feel free to use any frozen fruit you have on hand.

16 ounces frozen tropical fruit mix

8 ounces coconut water

8 ounces water

2 tablespoons chia seeds

2 scoops unflavored protein powder (40 grams of protein)

1. Combine the fruit, coconut water, water, chia seeds, and protein powder in a blender and process until combined. (If your blender is small, you can make this in two batches.)

2. Portion ¾ cup of smoothie into each of 6 glass jars and seal.

3. Refrigerate for up to 3 days or freeze for up to 2 months. To serve from frozen, thaw in the refrigerator overnight or enjoy frozen like a slushy.

INGREDIENT TIP: These smoothies make great freezer pops. Pour the mixture into ice pop molds and freeze for 6 hours.

PER SERVING: Calories: 95; Total fat: 2g; Total carbs: 14g; Sugar: 10g; Protein: 7g; Fiber: 3g; Sodium: 52mg

Green Goodness Smoothie

PREP TIME: 10 minutes

MAKES 6 SERVINGS / GLUTEN-FREE, NUT-FREE, STAGE 2, UNDER 10, VEGETARIAN

Eating your greens may not be easy after surgery, but drinking them is. This crisp green smoothie will give you all the benefits of a serving of vegetables, along with a burst of energy to get your day started. Pairing your greens with citrus, whether orange or lemon, will help with iron absorption, too. If you have any vegetables in your refrigerator that need to be used, such as cucumber, romaine lettuce, avocado, zucchini, or kale, add them. Any greens will work great.

3 cups baby spinach

1 cup chopped fresh parsley

1 cup light orange juice

1 cup water

1 cup frozen grapes or pineapple chunks

2 tablespoons flaxseed meal

3 scoops unflavored protein powder (10 grams per serving), divided

1. Combine the spinach, parsley, orange juice, and water in a blender. Blend until smooth. You may need to open the lid and push the greens into the liquid, because they can stick to the sides.

2. Add the grapes and flaxseed and continue to blend until smooth.

3. Portion ¾ cup of smoothie into each of 6 glass jars and seal.

4. Refrigerate for up to 2 days or freeze for up to 2 months. To serve from frozen, thaw in the refrigerator overnight.

5. Before serving, add ½ scoop of protein powder and give it a good shake or stir.

VARIATION: You can swap out the flaxseed meal with chia seeds, hemp seeds, peanut butter, or even cocoa powder.

PER SERVING: Calories: 92; Total fat: 1g; Total carbs: 12g; Sugar: 8g; Protein: 9g; Fiber: 2g; Sodium: 35mg

Chocolate Cherry Shake

PREP TIME: 10 minutes

MAKES 6 SERVINGS / 5-INGREDIENT, DAIRY-FREE, STAGE 1, UNDER 10, VEGETARIAN

This shake, which was inspired by chocolate-covered cherries, has a rich and intense flavor. You will feel like you are having dessert for breakfast, all while you are loading up on nutrients. Cocoa provides antioxidants, which can protect your cells and tissue from damage. It is believed that the higher percentage of cocoa or cacao, the greater the benefits. Cocoa is also rich in magnesium, which is linked to improved mood.

1 (16-ounce) bag frozen cherries

2 cups unsweetened vanilla almond milk

4 tablespoons unsweetened cocoa powder

2 tablespoons nut butter of choice

2 scoops unflavored protein powder (40 grams of protein)

1. Combine the cherries, almond milk, cocoa, nut butter, and protein powder in a blender. Blend until smooth.

2. Portion ¾ cup of smoothie into each of 6 glass mason jars and seal.

3. Refrigerate for up to 3 days or freeze for up to 3 months. To serve from frozen, thaw in the refrigerator overnight or enjoy frozen like a slushy.

INGREDIENT TIP: Cherry skin is thick, so this smoothie may have more texture than others. You can add more liquid if desired.

PER SERVING: Calories: 124; Total fat: 5g; Total carbs: 13g; Sugar: 7g; Protein: 10g; Fiber: 3g; Sodium: 50mg

Sweet Potato–Almond Smoothie

PREP TIME: 10 minutes

MAKES 6 SERVINGS / GLUTEN-FREE, STAGE 1, UNDER 10, VEGETARIAN

This drink is like fall in a cup, and it was inspired by my mom's Thanksgiving sweet potato recipe. No marshmallow-covered potatoes ever graced our table. Instead, sweet potatoes were topped with lemon juice, cinnamon, and nutmeg—flavors you'll find in this drink. The pairing of sweet and sour in this recipe will offer balance and satisfy your sweet tooth without a sugar rush or crash. Sweet potatoes are a complex carbohydrate that our bodies digest slowly. If you want to reduce the carbohydrates further, use butternut squash instead.

1 (10-ounce) bag frozen chopped sweet potatoes or butternut squash

2 cups unsweetened vanilla almond milk

Juice of 1 lemon

2 scoops unflavored protein powder (40 grams of protein)

2 tablespoons almond butter

1 teaspoon pumpkin pie spice

1. Combine the sweet potatoes, almond milk, and lemon juice in a blender. Blend until smooth; use a slotted spoon or tongs to remove any stringy fibers.

2. Add the protein powder, almond butter, and pumpkin pie spice and pulse until smooth.

3. Portion ¾ cup of the smoothie into each of 6 glass jars and seal.

4. Refrigerate for up to 3 days or freeze for up to 3 months. To serve from frozen, thaw in the refrigerator overnight or mash with a fork and enjoy semi-frozen.

INGREDIENT TIP: To use fresh sweet potatoes instead of frozen, poke a few holes in them with a fork, wrap them in paper towels, and microwave for 4 to 5 minutes. Flip the potatoes over and microwave for another 3 to 5 minutes (depending on the size), until soft. Scoop out the flesh and use or freeze as needed.

PER SERVING: Calories: 126; Total fat: 4g; Total carbs: 13g; Sugar: 2g; Protein: 9g; Fiber: 3g; Sodium: 65mg

Savory Gazpacho Shake

PREP TIME: 10 minutes

MAKES 6 SERVINGS / GLUTEN-FREE, NUT-FREE, VEGETARIAN, UNDER 10

Gazpacho is a dish that originated in Spain and consists of blended raw vegetables, often with tomatoes as a base. You can make this with any variety of tomato, such as Roma, beefsteak, grape, or cherry. Just make sure the tomatoes are ripe and ready to eat, because that will affect sweetness and acidity. As for the onion, I suggest waiting until 3 months after surgery to include it, because onions have a pungent flavor and may cause some stomach discomfort.

5 cups diced ripe tomatoes

1 cucumber, peeled and sliced

1 small red or yellow bell
  pepper, chopped

2 cups low-sodium vegetable juice

½ small sweet onion (optional)

4 tablespoons chopped fresh parsley

2 tablespoons chopped fresh cilantro
  (optional)

2 tablespoons olive oil

Juice of 1 lemon

6 scoops unflavored protein powder
  (20 grams of protein per serving),
  divided

1. Combine the tomatoes, cucumber, bell pepper, vegetable juice, sweet onion (if using), parsley, cilantro (if using), oil, and lemon juice in a blender or food processor. Blend until smooth.

2. Portion ¾ cup of the gazpacho into each of 6 airtight containers and seal.

3. Refrigerate for up to 4 days or freeze for up to 6 months. To serve from frozen, thaw in the refrigerator overnight.

4. To serve, add 1 scoop of protein powder and shake with a shaker ball before drinking.

VARIATION: You can make leftovers into a hot soup, if preferred. Simmer in a medium pot on the stovetop until heated through. Add cooked quinoa or farro and top with some avocado for extra protein.

PER SERVING: Calories: 164; Total fat: 6g; Total carbs: 12g; Sugar: 7g; Protein: 18g; Fiber: 3g; Sodium: 88mg

Chia Pudding

PREP TIME: 10 minutes, plus 16 hours to set

MAKES 6 SERVINGS / 5-INGREDIENT, GLUTEN-FREE, NUT-FREE, VEGETARIAN

This chia pudding is packed with protein, omega-3 fatty acids, fiber, and antioxidants, and it's also delicious—like dessert in a cup. You can make this from any flavor of ready-to-drink protein shake. Or, you can build your own by choosing any flavored protein powder. Some favorites from my clients are cookies and cream, caramel, and coffee. No need to limit yourself to just chocolate and vanilla. You can also replace regular milk with any nondairy milk alternative to make this a dairy-free dessert.

6 tablespoons chia seeds

3 cups low-fat milk or nondairy milk

2 scoops protein powder (40 grams of protein)

½ cup sliced fresh fruit (optional)

1. Portion 1 tablespoon of chia seeds into each of 6 glass mason jars.

2. In a medium bowl, mix together the milk and protein powder until all the powder has dissolved. Pour ½ cup of the milk mixture into each jar. Stir and cover each jar with plastic wrap.

3. Refrigerate for at least 16 hours to set. Store the pudding and fruit (if using) separately in the refrigerator for up to 5 days. You can freeze the pudding for up to 2 months after it has set. Thaw frozen pudding in the refrigerator overnight before serving.

4. Top with a few slices of fruit, like strawberries or bananas (if using), before serving.

INGREDIENT TIP: Adjust for preferred thickness by increasing or decreasing the amount of milk. Also, stirring midway will help make a thicker pudding.

PER SERVING: Calories: 154; Total fat: 7g; Total carbs: 14g; Sugar: 6g; Protein: 10g; Fiber: 5g; Sodium: 84mg

Easy Homemade Granola

PREP TIME: 10 minutes / **COOK TIME:** 20 minutes
MAKES 8 SERVINGS / GLUTEN-FREE, VEGETARIAN

You might be craving the crunchy and sweet combination of granola, but store-bought versions are often loaded with sugar and additives. This recipe, on the other hand, cuts the sugar and calories, so you can enjoy it without worry. It's perfect to sprinkle on top of Greek yogurt, puddings, or breakfast bowls that need a little more texture.

¼ cup sugar-free syrup
¼ cup coconut oil or olive oil
2 cups old-fashioned rolled oats
½ cup chopped nuts of choice
¼ teaspoon ground cinnamon or
  pumpkin pie spice

¼ teaspoon salt
3 to 4 drops low-calorie liquid sweetener
  (optional)
32 ounces low-fat plain Greek yogurt

1. Preheat the oven to 350°F. Line a baking sheet with parchment paper.

2. In a small bowl, mix the syrup and oil together.

3. In a large bowl, combine the oats and nuts, then slowly pour in the syrup-oil mixture, stirring constantly. Make sure the oats are evenly coated in the liquid.

4. Spread the oat mixture on the prepared baking sheet, and press down to create an even layer. Sprinkle the cinnamon and salt evenly over the mixture.

5. Bake for 20 minutes, shaking the pan once halfway through.

6. Remove the baking sheet from the oven, stir the granola, and let it cool completely. If it still looks a little wet, that's okay; it will continue to dry out as it cools.

7. Portion ¼ cup of granola into each of 8 airtight containers and seal.

8. Stir the sweetener into the yogurt, if using. Portion ½ cup of yogurt into 8 small storage containers.

9. Store the granola on the counter for up to 1 month, and refrigerate the yogurt for up to 1 week. Mix just before serving.

INGREDIENT TIP: Coconut oil solidifies at 75° F, so if you store it in a cool pantry, you may need to warm it up to return it to liquid.

PER SERVING: Calories: 250; Total fat: 13g; Total carbs: 24g; Sugar: 9g; Protein: 10g; Fiber: 3g; Sodium: 183mg

Crustless Tomato, Broccoli, and Mozzarella Quiche

PREP TIME: 15 minutes / **COOK TIME:** 50 minutes

MAKES 8 SERVINGS / GLUTEN-FREE, NUT-FREE, VEGETARIAN, STAGE 3

This quiche is reminiscent of the broccoli pie I grew up eating for Sunday brunch, except this version is much healthier. The modification not only drastically reduces carbs, but also makes a filling, gluten-free meal. Slow-digesting veggies, such as broccoli, will help you stay full and satisfied for hours. The best part is that you can swap in any other combination of vegetables you prefer, like onions, peppers, zucchini, mushrooms, or spinach. Top with a different cheese, and you'll have created a completely new dish.

Nonstick cooking spray

2 teaspoons olive oil

2 garlic cloves, sliced

1 cup chopped broccoli florets

4 ripe tomatoes, chopped

6 large eggs

½ cup low-fat milk

1 cup shredded low-fat mozzarella cheese

Salt

Freshly ground black pepper

1. Preheat the oven to 350°F. Spray a high-sided 9-inch pie pan with cooking spray, or coat it with oil.

2. In a large pan, heat the oil over medium heat and sauté the garlic until golden. Add the broccoli and tomatoes and cook them down to release their moisture, about 5 minutes.

3. While the veggies cook, in a medium bowl, whisk together the eggs and milk.

4. Transfer the vegetables to the pan, and spread them out evenly. Pour in the egg mixture and top evenly with mozzarella cheese. Sprinkle with salt and pepper.

5. Bake for 45 to 50 minutes, until a toothpick inserted in the center comes out clean. Let cool completely.

6. Cut the quiche into 8 slices, place 1 slice in each of 8 airtight containers, and seal.

7. Refrigerate for up to 4 to 5 days, or wrap in aluminum foil, seal in a freezer bag, and freeze for up to 2 months. Reheat from the refrigerator in the microwave for 1 to 2 minutes. To reheat from the freezer, thaw in the refrigerator overnight, unwrap, and then microwave, or place the foil-wrapped quiche in a 350°F oven for 15 to 20 minutes.

VARIATION: You can use any leftover roasted vegetables or cooked chicken for this. Just skip to step 4.

PER SERVING: Calories: 130; Total fat: 8g; Total carbs: 5g; Sugar: 3g; Protein: 9g; Fiber: 1g; Sodium: 183mg

Zesty Fava Beans

PREP TIME: 10 minutes / **COOK TIME:** 1 hour

MAKES 8 SERVINGS / GLUTEN-FREE, STAGE 3, VEGAN

Inspired by a popular Middle Eastern dish, foul mudammas, this fiber- and protein-rich meal may open you up to a whole new world of breakfast choices. The lemon and garlic make this flavorful dish appealing in the early weeks after surgery (soft diet), and it's also satisfying as a side dish years later. This recipe uses dried, skinless fava beans, since they are available year-round and cut down on the prep time. Need to reduce cooking time further? Replace the favas with frozen or canned beans and skip the rehydrating process completely.

4½ cups water

1½ cups fava beans, split or blanched

1 teaspoon salt

½ teaspoon ground cumin

Juice of 1 large lemon

1 garlic clove, minced or mashed

1 cup chopped tomato, for serving

½ cup chopped fresh parsley, for serving

3 tablespoons olive oil, for serving

1. Rinse the beans. In a large saucepan, combine the water, beans, salt, and cumin over high heat. Bring to a boil. Then reduce the heat to low, cover, and simmer for 45 minutes.

2. When the beans are soft, mash with a large fork or potato masher.

3. In a small bowl, mix the lemon juice and the garlic. Add to the cooked beans and stir. Let cool.

4. Portion about ¾ cup into each of 6 airtight containers and seal. Store the tomato and parsley separately.

5. Refrigerate for up to 5 days. Reheat the beans in the microwave 30 seconds at a time, stirring in between.

6. To serve, add 1 heaping tablespoon of the tomato-parsley mixture on top of the beans and drizzle with 1 teaspoon of oil.

> **INGREDIENT TIP:** Fava beans are very nutritious. If you have more time, buy them fresh. They need to be peeled, cooked, and shelled. It is not difficult, and the process may even be relaxing.

PER SERVING: Calories: 73; Total fat: 5g; Total carbs: 6g; Sugar: 3g; Protein: 2g; Fiber: 2g; Sodium: 300mg

Low-Carb Breakfast Burritos

PREP TIME: 10 minutes / **COOK TIME:** 20 minutes

MAKES 6 SERVINGS / NUT-FREE

This breakfast burrito will make you want to wake up in the morning. Unlike most store-bought options, this burrito is packed with protein and low in carbs, thanks to the high-protein wrap—I recommend Loven Fresh (12 grams protein) or Mission Protein (7 grams protein) brands. Plus, it's a flavorful and filling breakfast to easily grab on the go. Bell peppers and sausage are a great combination that will have you savoring every bite.

Nonstick cooking spray

1 bell pepper, diced

1 medium onion, diced

3 breakfast sausage links (extra-lean or reduced-fat)

6 large eggs

3 tablespoons low-fat milk

6 high-protein wraps

2 cups shredded Colby and Monterey Jack cheese blend

Salt

Freshly ground black pepper

1. Place a large pan over medium heat and spray it with cooking spray. Add the pepper and onion and cook for about 10 minutes, until tender. Set aside to cool on a plate.

2. In the same pan, cook the sausage until it's heated through, about 5 minutes, or until it registers 160°F on an instant-read thermometer. Transfer the sausage to a paper-towel-lined plate to cool.

3. Reduce the heat to low. In a large bowl, whisk together the eggs and milk. Pour the egg mixture into the pan and cook, stirring frequently, until the eggs are scrambled, 3 to 4 minutes.

4. Cut the breakfast sausage into small pieces.

5. To assemble the burritos, lay 1 wrap on top of each of 6 pieces of aluminum foil. Sprinkle 1 ounce of cheese onto each wrap, then evenly divide the eggs and sausage between the wraps. Top with a thin layer of cooled peppers and onions. Fold in the sides of each wrap, roll them up, and cover tightly with foil.

6. Refrigerate for up to 4 days or freeze for up to 3 months. To reheat from the refrigerator, remove the foil and heat in the microwave for 1 to 1½ minutes. To reheat from the freezer, remove the foil and wrap in a paper towel. Heat for 3 minutes in the microwave, flip, then cook for another 2 minutes.

INGREDIENT TIP: It's important to wait for the ingredients to cool; adding hot ingredients to the wrap will make the burritos soggy.

PER SERVING: Calories: 440; Total fat: 24g; Total carbs: 30g; Sugar: 3g; Protein: 24g; Fiber: 2g; Sodium: 413mg

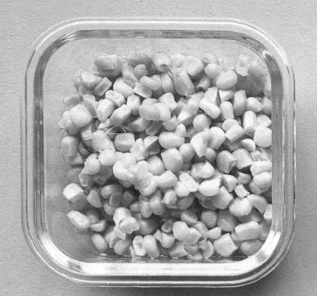
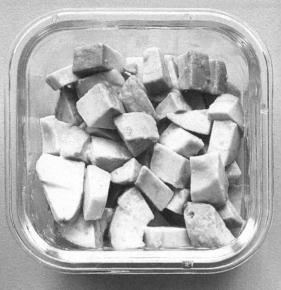

CHICKEN TORTILLA SOUP **118**

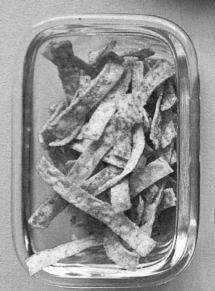
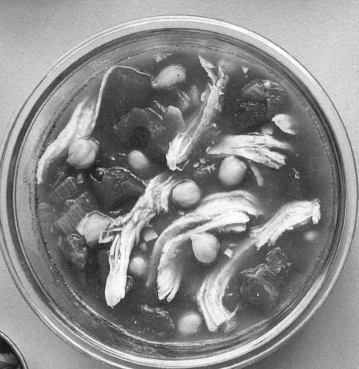
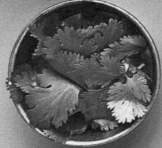

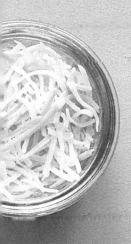

CHAPTER SIX

Soups and Stews

FRENCH ONION SOUP **116**

CHICKEN TORTILLA SOUP **118**

SLOW-COOKED BEEF STEW **120**

SEAFOOD CHOWDER **122**

TOMATO, LENTIL, AND VEGETABLE STEW **124**

BUTTERNUT SQUASH SOUP **125**

FRAGRANT CHICKEN CURRY STEW **126**

French Onion Soup

PREP TIME: 15 minutes / **COOK TIME:** 50 minutes

MAKES 6 SERVINGS / NUT-FREE

This fabulous version of French onion soup doesn't require much time but is still rich in flavor. Baking the croutons and using less butter makes this healthier, and the bold beef broth and sweet onions create a savory liquid that enhances the flavor. Don't forget to top the liquid with the croutons. This will prevent your cheese from settling to the bottom and allow you to enjoy the nutty Swiss cheese flavor with each spoonful.

¼ cup unsalted butter

4 tablespoons olive oil, divided

4 cups sliced sweet onions

6 cups beef broth or Bone Broth (page 29)

1 teaspoon dried thyme

Pinch salt

Pinch freshly ground black pepper

2 to 3 ounces day-old bread, multigrain or baguette

4 ounces Swiss cheese, sliced

3 scoops unflavored protein powder (60 grams of protein)

1. In a large stock pot, melt the butter and 2 tablespoons of oil over medium heat. Add the onions, stir, and cook for about 10 minutes, until the onions are soft and translucent.

2. Add the broth, thyme, salt, and pepper; simmer for 30 minutes.

3. Preheat the oven to 375°F.

4. Cut the bread into bite-size cubes, then place them in a large bowl and toss with the remaining 2 tablespoons of oil. Season with more salt and pepper.

5. Spread the bread cubes out in an even layer on a baking sheet. Bake for 10 minutes or until the croutons are crispy and golden brown. Let cool.

6. Portion ¾ cup of soup into each of 6 airtight containers and seal. Divide the croutons among 6 resealable bags, removing the air from the bags.

7. Refrigerate the soup for up to 1 week or freeze for up to 4 months. Store the croutons separately in a cool, dry place. You can also freeze the croutons for up to 6 weeks and reheat them in a 300°F oven for 3 to 5 minutes. Reheat the soup in the microwave for 2 minutes.

8. To serve, add the croutons and top with a slice of Swiss cheese. (If you would like to heat the cheese, place the soup in an oven-safe ramekin on a baking sheet, and broil until the cheese bubbles and browns slightly.) Add ½ scoop of protein powder once the soup cools enough to drink (under 140°F), and stir with a fork.

INGREDIENT TIP: Unlike butter, extra-virgin olive oil will smoke at high heat. If the only olive oil you have is extra-virgin, use canola oil instead.

PER SERVING: Calories: 332; Total fat: 22g; Total carbs: 18g; Sugar: 6g; Protein: 15g; Fiber: 1g; Sodium: 159mg

Chicken Tortilla Soup

PREP TIME: 20 minutes / **COOK TIME:** 45 minutes

MAKES 6 SERVINGS / GLUTEN-FREE

You may think soup is best on a cold day. However, this one is fabulous on a hot day, too. The zesty lime and heat from the chili powder remind me of countries with hot climates, like Mexico. This version is not as spicy as the traditional one, but you can add jalapeño or more cayenne if you are cleared to increase the heat in your dishes. Spicy food, which causes you to sweat, can help you feel cooler. So, remember to add this to your weekly meal prep when the temperatures rise.

3 tablespoons olive oil, divided

1 small onion, peeled and finely diced

4 garlic cloves, minced

1½ pounds boneless, skinless chicken breasts

4 cups low-sodium chicken broth or Bone Broth (page 29)

1 (14.5-ounce) can diced tomatoes

1 (15-ounce) can chickpeas, drained and rinsed

Juice of 1 lime

1 tablespoon chili powder

4 corn tortillas, cut into thin strips or store-bought baked tortilla strips

6 ounces shredded cheese blend, such as Mexican or cheddar

1. In a large stockpot, heat 2 tablespoons of oil over medium heat. Add the onion and sauté for 5 minutes, until it begins to soften.

2. Add the garlic and sauté for 1 to 2 minutes.

3. Add the chicken and cover with the broth. Then add the tomatoes and their juices, chickpeas, lime juice, and chili powder and bring to a boil.

4. Reduce the heat to low and simmer for 20 minutes or until the chicken's internal temperature reaches 165°F. Avoid overcooking or the chicken will get tough and chewy.

5. While the soup cooks, preheat the oven to 350°F.

6. In a medium bowl, place the tortilla strips with 1 tablespoon of oil and lightly coat. (You can skip this and the next step for store-bought tortilla strips.)

7. Lay them flat on a baking sheet and bake for 15 minutes, until crisped and lightly browned. Set aside to cool.

8. Once cooked, remove the chicken from the pot. Set aside to cool, and then shred it.

9. Portion 3 to 4 ounces of shredded chicken and ¾ cup of cooled broth into each of 6 airtight containers. Divide the tortilla strips among 6 airtight containers or storage bags.

10. Refrigerate the soup for 3 to 4 days or freeze up to 4 months. Store the tortilla strips on the counter for 1 week.

11. Reheat in the microwave for 1 to 2 minutes or on the stovetop until warm. Serve topped with tortilla strips and cheese.

VARIATION: You can also top this dish with cilantro, corn, diced avocado, or low-fat sour cream.

PER SERVING: Calories: 411; Total fat: 19g; Total carbs: 24g; Sugar: 5g; Protein: 37g; Fiber: 6g; Sodium: 282mg

Slow-Cooked Beef Stew

PREP TIME: 30 minutes / **COOK TIME:** 4 to 8 hours
MAKES 8 SERVINGS / DAIRY-FREE, NUT-FREE

Beef may be difficult to digest after surgery because of the collagen, but cooking it over low heat for a long time breaks down the tough connective tissues, allowing it to become tender. If you love beef, this cooking method will make the pre-surgery favorite enjoyable again. And this meal has so much richness, thanks to the browning process. You can skip the browning process if you prefer, but it impacts the flavor.

2 tablespoons olive oil

2 pounds beef stew meat (chuck roast), cut into 1-inch cubes

½ teaspoon salt

3½ cups beef stock, divided

4 carrots, chopped

1 onion, chopped

2 tablespoons tomato paste

2 tablespoons balsamic vinegar (optional)

2 garlic cloves, minced

2 bay leaves

Chopped fresh parsley or basil, for garnish (optional)

1. In a large sauté pan or Dutch oven, heat the oil over medium-high heat. Season the beef with salt and brown on each side, about 10 minutes. Transfer the meat to a slow cooker.

2. Add 1 cup of stock to the pan and stir to loosen any pieces of meat, then pour the liquid into the slow cooker. Add the remaining 2½ cups of stock to the slow cooker, along with the carrots, onion, tomato paste, vinegar (if using), garlic, and bay leaves.

3. Cook for 7 to 8 hours on low heat or 3 to 4 hours on high heat, until the meat is fork-tender.

4. Allow to cool overnight in the refrigerator. Remove the bay leaves.

5. Portion ½ cup of the stew into each of 8 airtight containers and seal.

6. Refrigerate for up to 5 days or freeze for up to 3 months. To reheat from frozen, defrost for 24 hours in the refrigerator, then reheat over low heat on the stovetop.

7. To serve, garnish with parsley or basil (if using).

INGREDIENT TIP: When cubing meat, remove larger pieces of fat, but keep some of it, because that helps keeps the meat tender.

VARIATION: To cook the stew in the oven, brown the meat in an ovenproof pot or Dutch oven, and leave the meat in the pot. Add the stock, scrape up any brown bits, and then stir in the carrots, onion, tomato paste, vinegar, garlic, and bay leaves. Cover the pot and cook the stew in a 350° F oven for 2½ hours.

PER SERVING: Calories: 193; Total fat: 8g; Total carbs: 5g; Sugar: 3g; Protein: 25g; Fiber: 1g; Sodium: 261mg

Seafood Chowder

PREP TIME: 30 minutes / **COOK TIME:** 51 minutes

MAKES 8 SERVINGS / ONE POT

This heart-healthy version of chowder is creamy, delicious, and nutritious. There are two main ways to make a fish chowder, according to New England standards— with milk or with tomatoes. This recipe uses milk to provide more protein. However, unlike traditional varieties, this soup reduces the fat by swapping cream for fat-free milk. In addition, you can choose from a variety of fish. I listed a few below, but most firm fish will work.

2 teaspoons olive oil

1 large onion, diced

4 cups fat-free milk

1 cup peeled, diced potato

1 cup peeled, diced carrots

1 teaspoon salt

1 pound firm whitefish (such as cod, haddock, sea bass, mahi-mahi, or tilapia), cut into 1-inch pieces

1 cup peas or edamame

2 tablespoons cold water

1 tablespoon all-purpose flour

Fresh parsley, for garnish (optional)

1. In a 6-quart saucepan, heat the oil over medium heat. Add the onion and sauté until tender, about 6 minutes.

2. Add the milk, potato, carrots, and salt. Bring to a simmer, then reduce the heat to low, cover, and cook for about 30 minutes, until the potatoes are tender.

3. Using a slotted spoon, transfer most of the potatoes to a food processor or blender. Blend and return the smooth mixture to the pot. Add additional milk or water, if needed.

4. Add the fish and peas, then turn the heat back up to medium.

5. In a small bowl, mix the water and flour and add it to the saucepan.

6. Bring the soup back to a gentle boil, then reduce and simmer for another 10 to 15 minutes. The fish should flake easily.

7. Portion ½ cup of chowder into each of 8 airtight containers, let cool, and seal.

8. Refrigerate for up to 4 to 5 days or freeze for up to 3 months. To reheat from frozen, thaw in the refrigerator for 24 hours and then reheat on the stove until heated through, about 5 minutes. Serve garnished with parsley, if desired.

SUBSTITUTION: To further reduce the carbohydrates in this stew, replace the potato with cauliflower.

PER SERVING: Calories: 148; Total fat: 3g; Total carbs: 15g; Sugar: 8g; Protein: 16g; Fiber: 2g; Sodium: 541mg

Tomato, Lentil, and Vegetable Stew

PREP TIME: 10 minutes / **COOK TIME:** 4 hours

MAKES 8 SERVINGS / GLUTEN-FREE, NUT-FREE, ONE POT, STAGE 3, VEGAN

I love making lentil soups because no overnight soaking is required. They're found in many cuisines, including Indian, Moroccan, French, and Egyptian. And the mild earthy flavor they impart makes them open to different spices. You can use green lentils instead of brown, because they have a similar texture.

4 cups water

2 cups brown lentils, rinsed

2 cups chopped tomatoes

2 cups spinach

1 cup button or cremini mushrooms

6 garlic cloves, minced

3 low-sodium vegetable bouillon cubes

2 teaspoons curry powder

1 teaspoon ground turmeric

2 tablespoons olive oil (optional)

Juice of 1 lemon (optional)

1. In a slow cooker, combine the water, lentils, tomatoes, spinach, mushrooms, garlic, bouillon, curry powder, and turmeric.

2. Cover and cook on low for 3 to 4 hours. For softer lentils, cook for 6 to 8 hours.

3. Portion 1 cup of stew into each of 8 airtight containers, let cool, and seal.

4. Refrigerate for up to 4 days or freeze for 6 months. Reheat on the stovetop or in the microwave in 1-minute intervals. To reheat from frozen, thaw in the refrigerator overnight.

5. To serve, drizzle with 1 teaspoon of oil and 1 teaspoon of lemon juice (if using).

INGREDIENT TIP: Want to thicken the soup? Remove about 1 cup of liquid an hour before the soup is done and mix it with 2 tablespoons of flour. Pour the mixture back into the slow cooker. Or, add 2 tablespoons of tomato paste.

PER SERVING: Calories: 193; Total fat: 1g; Total carbs: 35g; Sugar: 3g; Protein: 13g; Fiber: 6g; Sodium: 28mg

Butternut Squash Soup

PREP TIME: 25 minutes / **COOK TIME:** 3 hours or 45 minutes
MAKES 8 SERVINGS / ONE POT, STAGE 1, VEGAN

This soup is rich in beta-carotene and vitamins A, C, and E. Tofu adds protein and keeps it vegan, but you could use Greek yogurt instead if you like.

1 large butternut squash, peeled and cubed (about 6 cups)

3 large carrots, peeled and chopped

1 large sweet onion, quartered

3 cups vegetable broth

1 cup coconut milk, boxed, not canned (optional)

¼ teaspoon ground cinnamon

¼ teaspoon ginger paste

⅛ teaspoon ground nutmeg

⅛ teaspoon chili powder

16 ounces extra-firm tofu, cut into 1-inch cubes

1. In a slow cooker, combine the squash, carrots, onion, broth, coconut milk (if using), cinnamon, ginger paste, nutmeg, and chili powder.

2. Cover and cook on high for 3 to 4 hours.

3. Blend the soup with an immersion blender, or let it cool and then blend it in a food processor.

4. Portion about ¾ cup of soup into each of 8 airtight containers and let cool. Add 2 ounces tofu to each container for refrigerator storage. If freezing, do not add tofu. Freeze the tofu separately, let it thaw, press it between paper towels, and reheat it separately in a pan. The texture will be firmer and more meat-like.

5. Refrigerate the soup for up to 4 days or freeze for up to 4 to 5 months. Reheat in a microwave-safe bowl, covered partially with a lid. Heat in 2-minute intervals, stirring in between.

INGREDIENT TIP: You can also make this on the stovetop. Bring the soup to a boil, then reduce the heat, cover, and simmer for 45 minutes.

PER SERVING: Calories: 124; Total fat: 4g; Total carbs: 19g; Sugar: 6g; Protein: 7g; Fiber: 4g; Sodium: 32mg

Fragrant Chicken Curry Stew

PREP TIME: 30 minutes / **COOK TIME:** 45 minutes
MAKES 8 SERVINGS / DAIRY-FREE, ONE POT

This dish is enjoyable from start to finish—from the fragrant aroma while cooking, to the nourishing satisfaction hours later. Many curries pack some heat, but in this recipe I replaced the traditional serrano pepper with a sweet bell pepper to help you avoid heartburn. However, if that is not a concern, feel free to use a serrano pepper or up the cayenne.

2 tablespoons olive oil

2 small onions, finely chopped

1 red bell pepper, chopped

4 garlic cloves, minced

1½ tablespoons mild curry powder

1 tablespoon ginger paste

¼ teaspoon ground cayenne pepper (optional)

1½ pounds boneless, skinless chicken breasts or thighs

1½ cups light canned coconut milk

1 cup low-sodium chicken broth or Bone Broth (page 29)

Chopped fresh cilantro, for garnish (optional)

1. In a large saucepan or Dutch oven, heat the oil over medium heat and sauté the onions and pepper until soft, about 5 minutes.

2. Reduce the heat to low and add the garlic, curry powder, ginger, and cayenne (if using); stir for 1 to 2 minutes, until the aroma of spices is released.

3. Transfer the onions and pepper to a plate, then add the chicken to the pan. Brown the chicken on the outside, about 1 minute per side. You do not have to cook it all the way through.

4. Add the coconut milk, broth, and pepper-onion mixture to the pan, and stir to help deglaze the pan.

5. Cook on low heat, uncovered, for 20 minutes. Remove a piece of chicken and check that the internal temperature has reached 165°F.

6. Portion ½ cup of stew into each of 6 airtight containers, let cool, and seal.

7. Refrigerate for up to 3 days or freeze for up to 4 months. Reheat in the microwave for 1 minute, stir, and add 30 seconds at a time, as needed.

8. To serve, garnish with cilantro (if using).

VARIATION: Cooking the chicken on the stovetop gives it more texture, but you can also combine the ingredients in a slow cooker and cook the curry on high for 3 to 4 hours. This is also great served over cauliflower rice.

PER SERVING: Calories: 207; Total fat: 13g; Total carbs: 5g; Sugar: 1g; Protein: 18g; Fiber: 1g; Sodium: 87mg

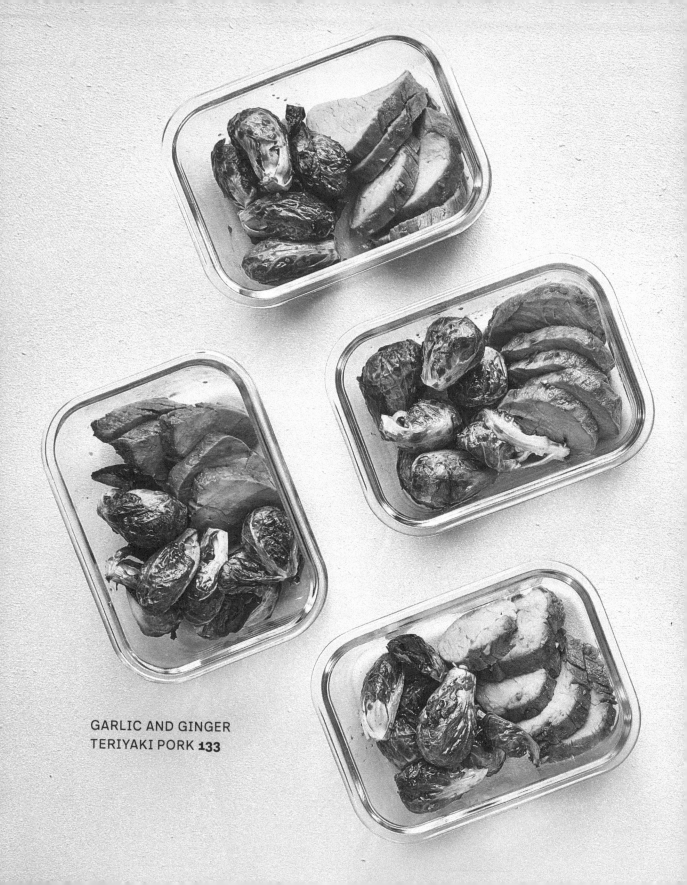

GARLIC AND GINGER
TERIYAKI PORK **133**

Healthy Mains

EGG ROLL BOWL **130**

BARBECUE CHICKEN TENDERS **132**

GARLIC AND GINGER TERIYAKI PORK **133**

CAULIFLOWER FRIED RICE WITH SHRIMP **135**

SHRIMP PARMIGIANA **137**

CHICKEN CORDON BLEU **139**

CHICKEN PESTO ROLL-UPS **141**

BUTTERY LEMON CODFISH **143**

HONEY SALMON WITH TANGY TZATZIKI SAUCE **144**

STEAK AND VEGGIE STIR-FRY **145**

Egg Roll Bowl

PREP TIME: 20 minutes / **COOK TIME:** 15 minutes
MAKES 4 SERVINGS / GLUTEN-FREE, NUT-FREE

Eating your vegetables is rarely this fun. Cutting the vegetables into a lovely julienne makes them more visually appealing and also helps reduce the cooking time, allowing them to maintain a slightly crunchy texture, which works well alongside the meat. Ground pork has a distinctive flavor that works well for this recipe; however, you can swap it for lean ground turkey if you prefer. Because finding lean ground pork can be a little more challenging, I added a simple step to reduce the fat. It is worth the effort; your stomach will thank you.

1 pound lean ground pork

1 tablespoon sesame oil

1 head cabbage, thinly sliced

1 to 2 tablespoons water

3 carrots, julienned

1 large zucchini, julienned

2 scallions, both white and green parts, julienned and divided

3 tablespoons soy sauce

2 garlic cloves, minced

1 teaspoon grated fresh ginger or paste

4 large eggs (optional)

1. In a large, deep sauté pan, cook the pork over low heat for 4 to 5 minutes, stirring as it cooks to release the liquid, until it is cooked through.

2. Once cooked through, use a slotted spoon to place the meat between paper towels. Blot off the oil. Remove the liquid and fat from the pan and wipe the pan.

3. In the pan, heat the sesame oil over medium heat. Toss in the cabbage and cook for 5 to 8 minutes. Stir frequently, until desired tenderness. Add the water to help cook it down and not stick to the pan.

4. Add the carrots, zucchini, white parts of the scallions, soy sauce, garlic cloves, and ginger. Continue to stir for 3 to 4 minutes. Turn off the heat and let cool.

5. Portion 3 ounces of pork, 1 cup of cabbage mixture, and 1 tablespoon of the green parts of the scallions into each of 4 airtight containers.

6. Refrigerate for up to 4 days or freeze for up to 3 months. To reheat, thaw first in the refrigerator, then add to a lightly greased sauté pan. Cook over medium heat for about 5 minutes.

7. Once the mixture is hot, create a well in the middle of the pan. Crack an egg (if using) in the center, cook it thoroughly, then mix well.

INGREDIENT TIP: Julienne is a technique of cutting vegetables into ⅛-inch-long strips. You can also use a Y-shaped peeler or grater if you're short on time.

PER SERVING: Calories: 256; Total fat: 9g; Total carbs: 19g; Sugar: 10g; Protein: 29g; Fiber: 7g; Sodium: 807mg

Barbecue Chicken Tenders

PREP TIME: 15 minutes / COOK TIME: 38 minutes
MAKES 8 SERVINGS / DAIRY-FREE, GLUTEN-FREE, NUT-FREE

For a long time, I thought barbecue sauce was just spicy ketchup. Wow, was I wrong! I was thrilled to learn how many ways this condiment can be created—using berries or cherries to enhance sweetness or vinegars and Worcestershire sauce for tanginess. This recipe is on the milder side of the heat scale but provides a bold flavor to jazz up your chicken.

1 (10-ounce) can diced tomatoes with green chiles

⅓ cup tomato paste

¼ cup apple cider vinegar

4 tablespoons honey

2 tablespoons gluten-free Worcestershire sauce

2 tablespoons honey mustard

1 tablespoon chili powder

2 tablespoons olive oil

2 pounds (½-inch-thick) chicken tenders

1. In a large saucepan, combine the tomatoes and their juices, tomato paste, vinegar, honey, Worcestershire sauce, honey mustard, and chili powder over low heat. Simmer the sauce for about 30 minutes.

2. In a large skillet, heat the oil over medium heat. Add the chicken, leaving space between each tender. Cook for 3 to 4 minutes, flip, and cook 3 to 4 minutes on the other side, or until a thermometer reaches 165°F.

3. Remove and let cool, then slice the chicken into long 1-inch strips.

4. Portion 3 to 4 ounces of chicken into each of 8 airtight containers. Spoon 4 tablespoons of cooled sauce over the chicken.

5. Refrigerate for up to 4 days or freeze for up to 3 months. Reheat in a skillet on the stovetop over medium heat, stirring with sauce, until heated through.

INGREDIENT TIP: If the chicken tenders are thicker than ½ inch, pound them with a mallet to thin them out before cooking.

PER SERVING: Calories: 210; Total fat: 6g; Total carbs: 14g; Sugar: 11g; Protein: 26g; Fiber: 1g; Sodium: 320mg

Garlic and Ginger Teriyaki Pork

PREP TIME: 5 minutes, plus at least 30 minutes to marinate / **COOK TIME:** 45 minutes
MAKES 8 SERVINGS / DAIRY-FREE, NUT-FREE, ONE POT

This dish is a staple in my home that everyone enjoys. Cooking the pork in a flavorful liquid ensures that it is tasty and tender every time. Making teriyaki sauce at home is easy and inexpensive—you may never buy a bottle of store-bought sauce again. You likely have most of the ingredients already, and you can use this sauce to marinate other proteins, like shrimp and chicken, as well. Not to mention, the flavors intensify with time and make this dish even better when it is reheated.

1 cup water

½ cup reduced-sodium soy sauce

¼ cup apple cider vinegar

4 tablespoons packed brown sugar

2 tablespoons grated fresh ginger or
 ginger paste

6 garlic cloves, minced

2 teaspoons sesame oil

2 pounds pork tenderloin, trimmed

2 cups Brussels sprouts, trimmed

1. In a large bowl, mix together the water, soy sauce, vinegar, brown sugar, ginger, garlic, and sesame oil.

2. Place the pork in a 9-by-13-inch baking dish, and pour the marinade over top. Cover the baking dish with aluminum foil and let the pork marinate in the refrigerator for at least 30 minutes or up to 3 hours.

3. Preheat the oven to 350°F.

4. Place the Brussels sprouts in the baking dish with the pork, cover with the foil again, and bake for 45 minutes to 1 hour, until the pork registers 145°F on an instant-read thermometer.

5. Let the pork cool, then slice it into thin medallions.

continued

6. Portion 3 to 4 ounces of pork and ¼ cup Brussels sprouts into each of 8 airtight containers or freezer bags; seal.

7. Refrigerate for up to 3 days or freeze for up to 3 months. To reheat from the freezer, thaw in the refrigerator overnight. Reheat in the microwave or on the stovetop.

INGREDIENT TIP: Standard soy sauce contains wheat. To make this gluten-free, use tamari instead.

PER SERVING: Calories: 184; Total fat: 4g; Total carbs: 11g; Sugar: 7g; Protein: 26g; Fiber: 1g; Sodium: 642mg

Cauliflower Fried Rice with Shrimp

PREP TIME: 20 minutes / **COOK TIME:** 15 minutes
MAKES 4 SERVINGS / DAIRY-FREE, NUT-FREE, ONE POT

There are numerous store-bought riced cauliflower options available, but I encourage you to make your own when you have time. Pulse small batches of cauliflower in the food processor to maintain texture and prevent overmixing. You could swap the shrimp for a soft protein like tofu if you've had surgery less than three months ago. As time passes and your portion sizes increase, you can mix in more vegetables, like broccoli, asparagus, mushrooms, onions, peas, or peppers, to help with fullness and satiety.

1 large head cauliflower

1 tablespoon sesame oil

1 pound fresh or frozen shrimp, peeled and deveined

1 cup frozen edamame

2 large carrots, shredded

¼ cup reduced-sodium soy sauce

2 large eggs, beaten

Scallions, both green and white parts, sliced (optional)

1. Cut the cauliflower into florets and remove the core. Process the florets in a food processor or dice into small pieces until the cauliflower resembles rice.

2. In a large sauté pan or wok, heat the oil over high heat and add the shrimp. Cook for 3 to 4 minutes, until the color turns pink. Remove from the pan and set aside to cool.

3. To the same skillet, add the edamame and carrots. Cook for 3 to 4 minutes, until tender. Stir frequently to prevent sticking.

4. Add the cauliflower rice and soy sauce. Continue to stir frequently for another 3 to 4 minutes, until tender.

5. Make a well in the center of the pan and add the eggs. Stir as the eggs scramble for 2 minutes and then mix thoroughly until cooked through.

continued

6. Portion the cauliflower and shrimp into 4 airtight containers, let cool, and seal.

7. Refrigerate for up to 4 days or freeze for up to 6 months. Reheat in the microwave in 30-second intervals, stirring in between to prevent the shrimp from becoming rubbery. Or, if using thawed shrimp, sauté on the stovetop with 1 to 2 tablespoons of water. Sprinkle scallions (if using) on top for another layer of flavor.

VARIATION: You can skip scrambling the eggs and instead top the reheated dish with a fried egg prior to serving.

PER SERVING: Calories: 270; Total fat: 10g; Total carbs: 20g; Sugar: 7g; Protein: 29g; Fiber: 7g; Sodium: 1041mg

Shrimp Parmigiana

PREP TIME: 30 minutes / **COOK TIME:** 15 minutes
MAKES 4 SERVINGS / NUT-FREE

Parmigiana might ordinarily conjure images of eggplant, tomato sauce, and cheese. However, I made the switch to shrimp and find this flavorful combination even more appealing—mostly because it cuts the prep time drastically. The shrimp also reduces the fat of this dish and provides much more protein, making this just as nutritious as it is delicious.

2 tablespoons olive oil

3 garlic cloves, chopped

1 (15-ounce) can tomato sauce

1 tablespoon Italian seasoning

Nonstick cooking spray

1 pound medium raw shrimp, peeled, deveined, and tails removed

2 large eggs

2 tablespoons water

½ cup panko bread crumbs

¼ cup grated Parmesan cheese

4 ounces part-skim mozzarella cheese, ⅛-inch slices

1. In a large saucepan, heat the oil over medium heat. Add the garlic and sauté until slightly brown, about 2 minutes.

2. Gently pour the tomato sauce into the saucepan, along with the Italian seasoning, and stir. Bring it to a gentle boil, then reduce the heat to low and simmer for 20 minutes, while you prep the shrimp. Cooking the sauce longer will reduce acidity and add sweetness.

3. Preheat the oven to 350°F. Cover a baking dish with foil and coat with cooking spray.

4. Butterfly the shrimp by slicing it lengthwise almost all the way through, creating 2 mirrored sides.

5. In a small bowl, whisk the eggs and water to combine. Add the bread crumbs and cheese to another shallow bowl.

6. Dip the shrimp into the eggs and then the bread crumbs.

continued

7. Place the coated shrimp in a single layer on the baking dish. Spray with a little more cooking spray, then bake for 10 to 12 minutes, until lightly browned and cooked through. Let cool.

8. Remove the sauce from heat and let cool.

9. In each of 4 airtight containers, layer 1 to 2 tablespoons of sauce, 2 to 3 ounces of shrimp, sauce again, and 1 ounce of mozzarella cheese.

10. Refrigerate for up to 3 days or freeze for up to 6 months. Wrap in foil and reheat in a 300°F oven until the cheese is melted, 12 to 15 minutes.

COOKING TIP: Keep a close eye on the cooking time, because overcooked shrimp can get rubbery and are difficult to digest.

PER SERVING: Calories: 330; Total fat: 17g; Total carbs: 14g; Sugar: 5g; Protein: 30g; Fiber: 2g; Sodium: 898mg

Chicken Cordon Bleu

PREP TIME: 30 minutes, plus 1 hour to set / **COOK TIME:** 30 minutes

MAKES 8 SERVINGS / NUT-FREE

Are you looking to upgrade the common ham-and-cheese roll-ups and take your chicken from bland to bold? If so, look no further than this delicious chicken recipe, which is so tasty you may think it's from a fancy French restaurant. Even more exciting is that this uses a solid protein instead of ground, allowing you to feel fuller longer as the years following your surgery pass.

4 boneless, skinless chicken breasts

4 ounces ham, thinly sliced

6 ounces sliced Swiss cheese, divided

Olive oil, for greasing

3 tablespoons light mayonnaise

4 tablespoons Dijon mustard, divided

1 cup panko bread crumbs

1 cup low-fat milk

1 tablespoon butter

1 tablespoon all-purpose flour

1. Place the chicken between two sheets of plastic wrap or in a large resealable bag. Using a mallet or rolling pin, flatten the chicken into a thin, even layer, about ¼ inch thick.

2. Remove the top layer of plastic wrap, and place 1 ounce of ham and 1 ounce of Swiss cheese on top of each flattened breast.

3. Roll up the chicken from the bottom, and then use the bottom piece of plastic from step 1 to wrap them tightly. Refrigerate for 1 to 2 hours. (This chilling step helps the chicken rolls keep their shape. If you like, use toothpicks to hold the rolls together, and skip to step 4.)

4. Preheat the oven to 350°F. Lightly grease a baking sheet and set aside.

5. Take the chicken roll-ups out of the refrigerator and peel off the plastic. In a small bowl, mix the mayonnaise with 2 tablespoons of the mustard. Spread the mayonnaise mixture over the top of the chicken roll-ups, then press bread crumbs into the mayonnaise mixture.

continued

6. Place the roll-ups on the prepared baking sheet. Bake, uncovered, for 30 to 40 minutes, or until the chicken reaches 165°F on an instant-read thermometer. Remove the chicken from the oven and let it cool, then slice the roll-ups into 2-inch pieces.

7. In a small bowl, heat the milk for 30 seconds in the microwave.

8. In a small saucepan, melt the butter over low heat, then whisk in the flour. Stir continuously for 2 minutes. Slowly add half the hot milk and continue to whisk. Add the remaining milk, remaining 2 tablespoons of mustard, and remaining 2 ounces of Swiss cheese. Whisk constantly for 3 to 4 minutes. The sauce will thicken as it cools.

9. Portion 2 to 3 pieces, depending on thickness, into each of 8 airtight containers; let cool and seal. Portion the sauce into resealable bags.

10. Refrigerate the chicken for up to 4 days, or freeze for up to 6 months. Refrigerate the sauce for up to 7 days or freeze for up to 3 months. (The sauce will separate if you freeze it; whisk it back together before serving.) If freezing the chicken, wrap individual portions in plastic wrap and then place them in storage containers. To reheat from the refrigerator, spoon 2 to 3 tablespoons of sauce onto a piece of foil. Lay the chicken on top, wrap it up in the foil, and bake in a 325°F oven for 10 to 15 minutes.

VARIATION: If you do not want to roll the chicken, you can cut a pocket into the center of the unpounded chicken breasts and stuff them with the ham and cheese. Close the pocket with toothpicks and bake for 30 to 35 minutes.

PER SERVING: Calories: 269; Total fat: 15g; Total carbs: 9g; Sugar: 2g; Protein: 25g; Fiber: 1g; Sodium: 445mg

Chicken Pesto Roll-Ups

PREP TIME: 20 minutes / **COOK TIME:** 35 minutes

MAKES 6 SERVINGS / GLUTEN-FREE

Basil, parsley, Parmesan, and pine nuts make such a lovely paste it should not be limited to pasta. I encourage you to add any protein of your liking to this pesto. Salmon is my personal favorite, but it also goes wonderfully with shrimp, turkey tenderloins, and even steak. The zesty lemon also brings out the freshness of the greens, and will help you absorb the iron from the spinach better.

2 cups baby spinach

½ cup fresh basil, stems removed

½ cup fresh parsley, stems removed

¼ cup vegetable broth

2 tablespoons lemon juice

3 tablespoons pine nuts

2 tablespoons olive oil, plus more for greasing

2 garlic cloves, peeled

3 tablespoons grated Parmesan cheese

1 to 1½ pounds chicken tenderloin

Salt

Freshly ground black pepper

1. Add the spinach, basil, parsley, broth, and lemon juice to a food processor and begin to blend. Scrape down the sides and continue to pulse.

2. Add the pine nuts, oil, and garlic and continue to pulse until you get a creamy texture. Stir in the Parmesan cheese. Set aside.

3. Preheat the oven to 350°F.

4. Place the chicken between two sheets of plastic wrap or in a heavy-duty large sealable bag. Using a mallet or rolling pin, flatten the chicken until it's about ¼-inch thick.

5. Spread the pesto evenly on one side of the chicken and roll from bottom to top. Repeat with each tenderloin.

6. Place the chicken in a lightly greased deep 9-by-13-inch baking dish, seam-side down. Season the chicken with salt and pepper, and bake uncovered for 30 to 35 minutes, or until the internal temperature reaches 165°F.

continued

7. Portion 3 to 4 ounces of chicken into each of 6 airtight containers, let cool, and seal.

8. Refrigerate for up to 4 days. To freeze, wrap individual portions tightly in plastic wrap, then place them in storage containers; store in the freezer for up to 3 months. To reheat, microwave for 30 seconds, flip over, and reheat for 30 seconds more. To reheat from frozen, thaw in the refrigerator overnight, then follow refrigerator reheating instructions.

INGREDIENT TIP: Pine nuts are more expensive than most other nuts. Store the remainder in storage containers in the freezer to add to their shelf life. You can also swap out pine nuts for toasted walnuts.

PER SERVING: Calories: 177; Total fat: 10g; Total carbs: 2g; Sugar: 0g; Protein: 19g; Fiber: 1g; Sodium: 116mg

Buttery Lemon Codfish

PREP TIME: 10 minutes / **COOK TIME:** 12 minutes

MAKES 8 SERVINGS / GLUTEN-FREE, NUT-FREE, ONE PAN, STAGE 3

Pacific and Atlantic cod provide heart-healthy omega-3 fatty acids, plus lean protein. The delicate fish has a slightly sweet flavor, and it pairs well with almost any vegetable; sweet bell peppers and zucchini noodles are my favorite.

1½ pounds cod fillets

2 teaspoons olive oil

Salt

Freshly ground black pepper

Juice of 2 lemons

2 tablespoons butter

1 lemon, thinly sliced

2 tablespoons chopped fresh parsley, for garnish

1. Preheat the oven to 400°F.

2. Coat the fish with the oil and season both sides with salt and pepper.

3. Add the fish to a deep 9-by-13-inch baking dish. Spoon the lemon juice over each piece. Top each piece with a thin pat of butter and a few lemon slices.

4. Bake for 10 to 12 minutes. The fish should flake apart when done.

5. Portion the cod into 8 airtight containers, let cool, and seal.

6. Refrigerate for up to 3 days or freeze for up to 3 months. Reheat on the stove-top until the fish is warmed through. To reheat from frozen, first thaw in the refrigerator for 24 hours.

7. To serve, garnish with parsley.

INGREDIENT TIP: If you wish to purchase a more sustainable variety of cod, choose Pacific and look for the blue MSC label.

VARIATION: This recipe also works with haddock, sea bass, mahi-mahi, or tilapia.

PER SERVING: Calories: 108; Total fat: 5g; Total carbs: 1g; Sugar: 0g; Protein: 15g; Fiber: 0g; Sodium: 89mg

Honey Salmon with Tangy Tzatziki Sauce

PREP TIME: 10 minutes / **COOK TIME:** 10 minutes

MAKES 4 SERVINGS / GLUTEN-FREE, NUT-FREE

This sweet and spicy salmon is quick to make and perfect for lunch or dinner, especially on a warm day. If you are not a fan of salmon, swap it out for some fresh tuna, frozen shrimp, or chicken breasts. Enjoy it cold over a bed of greens.

Juice of 2 large lemons, divided

3 tablespoons honey, divided

3 tablespoons olive oil, divided

⅛ teaspoon freshly ground black pepper

⅛ teaspoon ground cayenne pepper (optional)

1 pound salmon fillets, cut into 4-ounce pieces

1 small cucumber, peeled and diced

1 cup low-fat plain Greek yogurt

1 teaspoon finely chopped fresh or dried dill

1. In a small bowl, combine the juice from 1 lemon, 2 tablespoons of honey, 2 tablespoons of oil, black pepper, and cayenne (if using).

2. Coat the salmon with the honey-lemon mixture.

3. In a large saucepan, heat the remaining 1 tablespoon of oil over medium heat. Cook for 4 to 5 minutes per side, until it flakes easily with a fork.

4. In a medium bowl, combine the cucumber, yogurt, dill, and the remaining tablespoon of honey. Mix well.

5. Portion the salmon into 4 airtight containers or resealable bags, and portion the tzatziki sauce into 4 separate airtight containers or resealable bags.

6. Refrigerate for up to 4 days or freeze for up to 2 months. Whisk thawed tzatziki after freezing to reconstitute. Reheat the fish on a piece of aluminum foil, add 1 tablespoon of lemon juice, wrap it up, and bake in a 250°F oven for 15 to 20 minutes.

PER SERVING: Calories: 349; Total fat: 18g; Total carbs: 20g; Sugar: 18g; Protein: 26g; Fiber: 1g; Sodium: 95mg

Steak and Veggie Stir-Fry

PREP TIME: 8 minutes / **COOK TIME:** 15 minutes

MAKES 4 SERVINGS / DAIRY-FREE, NUT-FREE, ONE PAN

This stir-fry has a wonderful balance of all five tastes—sweet, salty, sour, bitter, and umami. Many of my clients find that creating dishes with multiple flavors increases satisfaction, preventing them from wanting to raid the refrigerator after their meal to counter one overpowering flavor. If you have time, do a little taste test game with the ingredients before cooking.

1 pound sirloin or flank steak, cut into thin strips

Salt

Freshly ground black pepper

1 tablespoon sesame or olive oil

2 tablespoons soy sauce

1 tablespoon brown sugar

1 small onion, chopped

1 cup sliced mushrooms

1 cup broccoli florets

Juice of 1 small orange

2 teaspoons grated fresh ginger or paste

1. Season the steak with salt and pepper. In a large skillet, heat the oil over medium heat and start to brown the meat for 2 to 3 minutes.

2. Add the soy sauce and brown sugar, and continue to stir until the meat browns, 1 to 2 minutes. Do not overcook as this will make meat tough. Set aside to cool.

3. In the same skillet, combine the onion, mushroom, broccoli, orange juice, and ginger and cook for about 5 minutes. Slightly undercook the vegetables, because this will give the dish a better texture after reheating.

4. Portion 3 ounces of steak and 1 cup of vegetables into each of 4 airtight containers, let cool, and seal.

5. Refrigerate for up to 4 days. Freezing is not recommended. Reheat over low to medium heat in a skillet that has been sprayed with cooking oil.

INGREDIENT TIP: Cut the meat against the grain (perpendicular to the fibers) to improve tenderness. Alternately, ask a butcher to do it for you.

PER SERVING: Calories: 226; Total fat: 9g; Total carbs: 9g; Sugar: 6g; Protein: 26g; Fiber: 1g; Sodium: 545mg

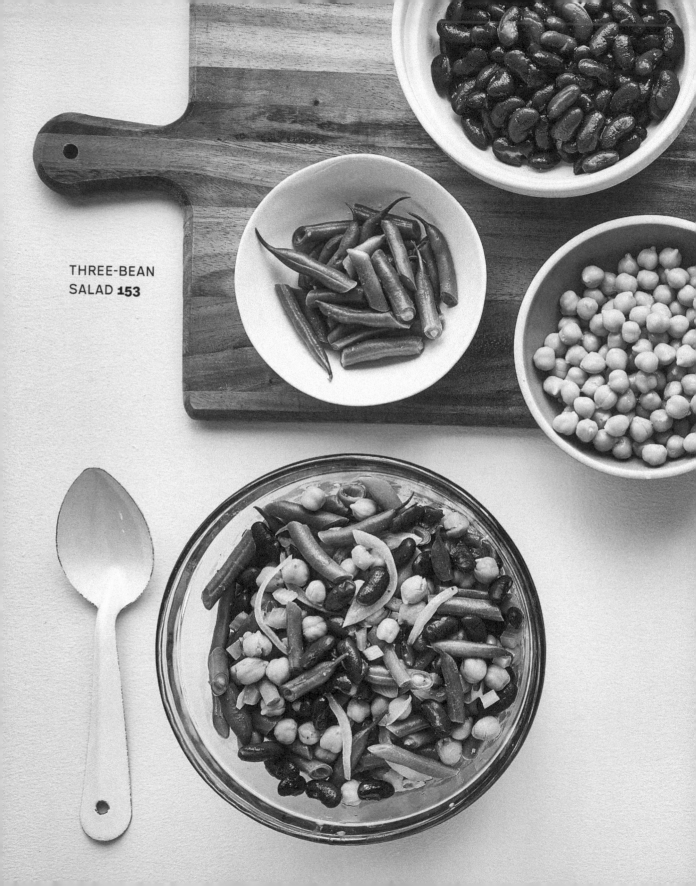

THREE-BEAN
SALAD **153**

CHAPTER EIGHT

Sweets and Snacks

AVOCADO CHOCOLATE MOUSSE **148**

DOUBLE CHOCOLATE HUMMUS **149**

CINNAMON APPLE "PIE" **150**

MANGO YOGURT POPS **152**

THREE-BEAN SALAD **153**

TURKEY-STUFFED MUSHROOMS **155**

CRUNCHY CABBAGE AND CARROT SLAW **157**

SPICY CHICKEN SALAD **158**

Avocado Chocolate Mousse

PREP TIME: 10 minutes

MAKES 6 SERVINGS / GLUTEN-FREE, STAGE 2, UNDER 10

Chocolate mousse is often a rich dessert made with heavy cream, making it high in saturated fat and cholesterol. This heart-healthy version is also rich, thanks to the creamy avocado. Avocado has healthy fats and 13 grams of fiber per fruit.

2 large ripe avocados, pitted and peeled

½ cup almond milk, warmed

½ cup no-sugar-added dark chocolate (such as Lily's), melted

½ cup dark brewed coffee (optional)

¼ cup unsweetened cocoa powder

1 scoop vanilla or chocolate protein powder (20 grams of protein)

1 tablespoon vanilla extract

⅛ teaspoon salt

1. Combine the avocados, almond milk, dark chocolate, coffee (if using), cocoa powder, protein powder, vanilla, and salt in a food processor; blend until smooth, scraping down the sides as needed. If the mousse seems too thick, add more almond milk, 1 tablespoon at a time, blending between additions. The mousse will thicken as it chills.

2. Portion the mousse into 6 glass jars or popsicle molds.

3. Refrigerate for up to 5 days or freeze for up to 3 months. Serve as is or with fruit on top, like berries or banana slices.

> **INGREDIENT TIP:** To help ripen avocados, lay them flat on the counter and don't pile anything on top. Check daily. Once the avocados are ripe, store them in the refrigerator until you're ready to use them.

PER SERVING: Calories: 182; Total fat: 14g; Total carbs: 11g; Sugar: 1g; Protein: 6g; Fiber: 7g; Sodium: 71mg

Double Chocolate Hummus

PREP TIME: 10 minutes

MAKES 8 SERVINGS / GLUTEN-FREE, VEGETARIAN, UNDER 10

If someone questions whether hummus can pass for dessert, my answer is: absolutely. This is a wonderfully sweet way to boost your protein and fiber. Use it as a dip, or spread it on a rice cake and top with fruit slices. You can even enjoy it on its own, just like yogurt or pudding.

1 (15-ounce) can white beans (great northern or navy)

¼ cup sugar-free syrup

2 tablespoons smooth peanut butter or almond butter

¼ cup unsweetened cocoa powder

1 teaspoon vanilla extract

⅛ teaspoon salt

1 scoop (30 grams) chocolate protein powder

2 tablespoons water, plus more as needed

1. Combine the beans, sugar-free syrup, and nut butter in a food processor. Pulse until smooth.

2. Add the cocoa powder, vanilla, and salt and continue to blend until everything is mixed in well, scraping down the sides as needed.

3. Add the protein powder and water and blend until smooth. Add additional water, 1 tablespoon at a time, to create your desired consistency.

4. Portion ¼ cup of the hummus into each of 8 airtight containers and seal.

5. Refrigerate for up to 5 days.

VARIATION: You can use almost any bean that you have in your pantry for this hummus; next time, try chickpeas or black beans.

PER SERVING (¼ CUP): Calories: 97; Total fat: 3g; Total carbs: 13g; Sugar: 5g; Protein: 7g; Fiber: 0g; Sodium: 75mg

Cinnamon Apple "Pie"

PREP TIME: 15 minutes / **COOK TIME:** 45 minutes

MAKES 4 SERVINGS / GLUTEN-FREE, STAGE 3, VEGETARIAN

You may have heard the adage, "An apple a day keeps the doctor away." Well, unfortunately, raw apples, especially the skins, are actually difficult to tolerate after surgery. This delicious and nutritious recipe will change that and will even remind you of apple pie as you indulge in the sweet cinnamon flavor. The best part is you won't feel guilty because there is no added sugar, only added protein. You can use any apple you have at home, but firmer apples such as Granny Smith, Honeycrisp, and Pink Lady do a great job at holding their texture.

Nonstick cooking spray

3 large apples, peeled, cored, and sliced

2 tablespoons lemon juice

½ cup old-fashioned rolled oats

¼ cup unsweetened almond milk

½ scoop vanilla protein powder (20 grams protein/scoop)

1 tablespoon butter, melted

1 teaspoon ground cinnamon

¼ teaspoon ground nutmeg

1. Preheat the oven to 325°F. Spray 4 ramekins with cooking spray.

2. In a large bowl, toss the apple slices with lemon juice, then place them in the ramekins in a circular pattern. Spritz the apples with nonstick cooking spray.

3. Place the ramekins on a baking sheet, transfer them to the oven, and bake for 30 minutes, until the apples are soft. You can test tenderness with a fork.

4. While the apples are baking, in a medium bowl, combine the oats, almond milk, protein powder, butter, cinnamon, and nutmeg. Mix well and let it sit to absorb the liquid.

5. Remove the apples from the oven, spread a layer of the oat mixture on top, and bake for 15 more minutes. Remove the desserts from the oven; let cool completely.

6. Cover the ramekins with plastic wrap and store them in the refrigerator for up to 5 days. To freeze the pies, remove them from the ramekins, wrap them in plastic wrap, and place them in a resealable plastic bag; they will keep in the freezer for up to 3 months.

7. Reheat in the microwave for 30 seconds. To reheat from frozen, thaw in the refrigerator overnight, then reheat.

INGREDIENT TIP: Top with Greek yogurt for extra protein.

PER SERVING: Calories: 178; Total fat: 4g; Total carbs: 32g; Sugar: 18g; Protein: 6g; Fiber: 6g; Sodium: 38mg

Mango Yogurt Pops

PREP TIME: 5 minutes

MAKES 4 SERVINGS / 5-INGREDIENT, GLUTEN-FREE, STAGE 1, UNDER 10, VEGETARIAN

Once you make these high-protein frozen yogurt pops, you'll wonder why you ever bought the store-bought version. Not only are these higher in protein, but they are so much less expensive. You can easily replace the mango with your favorite frozen fruit. If you enjoy texture in your pops, add fruit pieces into the mixture before spooning them into the molds. You can also make this dairy-free by using coconut yogurt.

8 ounces frozen mango chunks

1 cup low-fat plain Greek yogurt

1 scoop unflavored protein powder (equal to 20 grams of protein/scoop)

⅓ cup low-fat milk

1. Combine the mango, yogurt, protein powder, and milk in a food processor and blend until smooth.

2. Using a spoon, portion the mango mixture into 4 popsicle molds.

3. Cover and freeze for at least 6 hours or up to 6 months.

INGREDIENT TIP: Use plain protein powder so the flavor of the fruit will shine through.

PER SERVING: Calories: 100; Total fat: 2g; Total carbs: 14g; Sugar: 13g; Protein: 8g; Fiber: 1g; Sodium: 61mg

Three-Bean Salad

PREP TIME: 30 minutes / **COOK TIME:** 25 minutes

MAKES 4 SERVINGS / GLUTEN-FREE, NUT-FREE, STAGE 3, VEGAN

Beans are a great source of protein and fiber, but many people are afraid to eat them after surgery, due to the possibility that the legumes will cause bloating. This is due to the indigestible carbohydrates, known as oligosaccharides, that beans contain. Luckily, there are some simple ways to reduce the gassy effect of foods—soaking, rinsing, and cooking. This will help you enjoy beans more often and is worth the extra time.

½ onion, thinly sliced, soaked in cold water for 30 minutes

¼ cup olive oil, divided

1 (15-ounce) can no-sodium-added green beans, drained

1 cup canned no-sodium-added chick-peas, drained and rinsed

1 cup canned no-sodium-added kidney beans, drained and rinsed

1 celery stalk, finely chopped

½ cup water

⅓ cup apple cider or red wine vinegar

½ teaspoon celery seeds (optional)

⅛ teaspoon freshly ground black pepper

1. Drain and pat the soaked onion dry with paper towels.

2. In a medium saucepan, heat 1 tablespoon of oil over medium-high heat. Sauté the onion for 10 to 12 minutes, until soft.

3. Add the green beans, chickpeas, kidney beans, celery, water, and vinegar to the saucepan with the onions. Bring the mixture to a gentle boil, then reduce the heat to low and simmer for 10 minutes.

4. Remove the pan from the heat, add the celery seeds (if using) and pepper, and let the mixture cool.

5. Portion ¾ cup of salad into each of 4 airtight containers and seal.

continued

6. Refrigerate for up to 5 days or freeze for up to 1 month. If freezing, be sure to drain excess liquid to help reduce texture change. Thaw overnight in the refrigerator. You may need to season again with vinegar and spices, because the salad will lose some flavor in the freezer.

INGREDIENT TIP: Add the entire cans of chickpeas and kidney beans if you want to increase the servings.

PER SERVING: Calories: 273; Total fat: 15g; Total carbs: 27g; Sugar: 4g; Protein: 9g; Fiber: 8g; Sodium: 15mg

Turkey-Stuffed Mushrooms

PREP TIME: 30 minutes / **COOK TIME:** 20 minutes
MAKES 5 SERVINGS / NUT-FREE, STAGE 3

Stuffed mushrooms are the appetizer I always look forward to at parties, so I set out to create a recipe that is healthier than the traditional high-fat versions. With a few minor changes, I significantly reduced the amount of fat and calories in my take on the cocktail party staple. Don't wait for a special occasion. Enjoy these often as a snack anytime you like.

15 to 20 small mushrooms, such as
 button or cremini
1 tablespoon olive oil
4 ounces extra-lean ground turkey

4 garlic cloves, minced
¼ cup plain or panko bread crumbs
2 tablespoons grated Parmesan cheese
1 tablespoon dried parsley

1. Preheat the oven to 375°F. Line a baking sheet with parchment paper or brush it with oil.

2. Remove the stems from the mushrooms and set the caps aside. Rinse the stems, pat them dry, and chop them roughly.

3. In a large skillet, heat the oil over medium heat. Add the turkey, chopped mushroom stems, and garlic, and stir to combine.

4. Cook until the turkey is no longer pink, 7 to 10 minutes. Remove the skillet from the heat and drain any extra liquid.

5. Stir the bread crumbs, Parmesan, and parsley into the turkey-mushroom mixture.

6. Clean and dry the mushroom caps with a paper towel. Fill each cap with the turkey mixture, then place them on the prepared baking sheet. Bake for 15 to 18 minutes.

7. Portion 3 to 4 mushrooms into each of 5 airtight containers, let cool, and seal.

continued

8. Refrigerate for up to 5 days. Do not freeze. Reheat in the microwave at 30-second intervals until warm.

COOKING TIP: Though I don't recommend freezing the baked stuffed mushrooms, you can freeze the uncooked stuffed mushrooms and bake them up later. To do so, stuff the raw mushroom caps and flash-freeze them on a baking sheet for 1 to 2 hours, then transfer to airtight containers, separating layers with parchment paper; freeze for up to 2 months. To bake, place the frozen mushrooms directly in a 400°F oven for 15 minutes.

PER SERVING: Calories: 87; Total fat: 5g; Total carbs: 4g; Sugar: 1g; Protein: 6g; Fiber: 1g; Sodium: 74mg

Crunchy Cabbage and Carrot Slaw

PREP TIME: 15 minutes, plus at least 1 hour to chill

MAKES 8 SERVINGS / GLUTEN-FREE, NUT-FREE

This tangy and crunchy salad makes a wonderful snack or side for Cajun Chicken Sliders (page 88) or Lettuce-Wrap Shrimp Tacos with Chips and Guaca-mole (page 93). Unlike a mayo-based coleslaw, this slaw tastes better the longer you let it sit. However, it will lose some of its crunch as time goes on. If you like a little heat, add some cayenne pepper. If you prefer a sweeter taste, add an apple in addition to the jicama. If you can't find jicama, see the tip for swaps.

⅓ cup rice wine vinegar or white
   wine vinegar

4 teaspoons honey

Salt

Freshly ground black pepper

2 cups shredded green or red cabbage

1 cup grated carrot

1 small jicama, peeled and julienned

1. In a large bowl, whisk together the vinegar, honey, salt, and pepper.

2. Add the cabbage, carrot, and jicama and toss well. Cover and refrigerate for 1 to 2 hours.

3. Portion 1 cup of slaw into each of 4 airtight containers.

4. Store in the refrigerator for up to 5 days. Do not freeze.

INGREDIENT TIP: If jicama is unavailable, you can use a crisp green apple or rad-ishes instead.

PER SERVING: Calories: 43; Total fat: 0g; Total carbs: 10g; Sugar: 5g; Protein: 1g; Fiber: 3g; Sodium: 37mg

Spicy Chicken Salad

PREP TIME: 15 minutes, plus at least 30 minutes to marinate / **COOK TIME:** 10 minutes

MAKES 4 SERVINGS / DAIRY-FREE, GLUTEN-FREE, STAGE 3

Chicken breast is a great source of lean protein and can be seasoned in many different ways to keep it interesting. This recipe uses bold spices and citrus to amp up the flavors. The combination of lime juice and chili powder may make you think of a sizzling fajita. To make this a full meal instead of a snack, enjoy it in a low-carb wrap.

2 tablespoons freshly squeezed lime juice

2 tablespoons olive oil

½ tablespoon chili powder

½ teaspoon onion powder

⅛ teaspoon freshly ground black pepper

⅛ teaspoon cayenne pepper (optional)

1 pound boneless, skinless chicken breast (about 4 ounces each)

Nonstick cooking spray

1 red bell pepper, finely chopped (optional, omit if you aren't cleared for raw vegetables)

1 avocado, for serving (optional)

1. In a small bowl, mix together the lime juice, oil, chili powder, onion powder, pepper, and cayenne (if using).

2. Lay the chicken flat in a large glass baking dish, and apply a thin layer of the seasoning mixture on each side. Cover and let the chicken marinate in the refrigerator for at least 30 minutes or up to 3 hours.

3. Once the chicken is marinated, spray a large skillet with cooking spray and place it over high heat. Place the chicken in the skillet and cook for 4 to 5 minutes per side, until it's browned and registers 165°F on an instant-read thermometer.

4. Remove the skillet from the heat. Let the chicken cool, then dice it into small pieces and toss with the bell pepper (if using).

5. Portion 3 ounces of the salad into each of 4 airtight containers and seal.

6. Refrigerate for up to 4 days or freeze for up to 4 months.

7. To serve, mash ¼ avocado (if using) with each portion and mix.

VARIATION: You can swap out the avocado for 2-ounce mini packages of guacamole, such as Wholly Guacamole or Sabra.

PER SERVING: Calories: 190; Total fat: 9g; Total carbs: 1g; Fiber: 0g; Sugar: 0g; Protein: 25g; Sodium: 87mg

Measurement Conversions

VOLUME EQUIVALENTS	U.S. STANDARD	U.S. STANDARD (OUNCES)	METRIC (APPROXIMATE)
LIQUID	2 tablespoons	1 fl. oz.	30 mL
	¼ cup	2 fl. oz.	60 mL
	½ cup	4 fl. oz.	120 mL
	1 cup	8 fl. oz.	240 mL
	1½ cups	12 fl. oz.	355 mL
	2 cups or 1 pint	16 fl. oz.	475 mL
	4 cups or 1 quart	32 fl. oz.	1 L
	1 gallon	128 fl. oz.	4 L
DRY	⅛ teaspoon	–	0.5 mL
	¼ teaspoon	–	1 mL
	½ teaspoon	–	2 mL
	¾ teaspoon	–	4 mL
	1 teaspoon	–	5 mL
	1 tablespoon	–	15 mL
	¼ cup	–	59 mL
	⅓ cup	–	79 mL
	½ cup	–	118 mL
	⅔ cup	–	156 mL
	¾ cup	–	177 mL
	1 cup	–	235 mL
	2 cups or 1 pint	–	475 mL
	3 cups	–	700 mL
	4 cups or 1 quart	–	1 L
	½ gallon	–	2 L
	1 gallon	–	4 L

OVEN TEMPERATURES

FAHRENHEIT	CELSIUS (APPROXIMATE)
250°F	120°C
300°F	150°C
325°F	165°C
350°F	180°C
375°F	190°C
400°F	200°C
425°F	220°C
450°F	230°C

WEIGHT EQUIVALENTS

U.S. STANDARD	METRIC (APPROXIMATE)
½ ounce	15 g
1 ounce	30 g
2 ounces	60 g
4 ounces	115 g
8 ounces	225 g
12 ounces	340 g
16 ounces or 1 pound	455 g

Resources

BOOKS

Bariatric Fitness for Your New Life, by Julia Karlstad (Ulysses Press, 2018)

Bariatric Mindset Success: Live Your Best Life and Keep the Weight off After WLS, by Dr. Kristin Lloyd (CreateSpace, 2017)

My WLS Journey: 12 Week Food & Activity Tracker for Gastric Bypass Sleeve & Lapband Patients (SublimeLemons Notebooks, 2019)

A Pound of Cure: Change Your Eating and Your Life, One Step at a Time, by Dr. Matthew Woinor (CreateSpace, 2013)

Ultimate Gastric Sleeve Success: A Practical Patient Guide to Help Maximize Your Weight Loss Results, by Dr. Duc C. Vuong (HappyStance Publishing, 2013)

Weight Loss Surgery Does Not Treat Food Addiction, by Connie Stapleton, PhD (Mind Body Health Services, Inc., 2017)

COMMUNITY

- AmericanBariatrics.com
- Instagram @Dusty_Lost_300lbs
- GastricSleeve.com/forum

WEBSITES

- BariatricPal.com
- ObesityHelp.com
- ObesityCoverage.com

APPS AND PODCASTS

- Baritastic
- Calm
- MyFitnessPal
- Water Reminder
- *Real Talk with Suzi Shaw*
- *Reverse the Relapse After Weight Loss Surgery* with Georgie Beames
- *Weight Loss Surgery Podcast* by Reeger Cortell
- *Winning Through Weight Loss*

References

Aaron J. Dawes, Melinda Maggard-Gibbons, Alicia R. Maher, Marika J. Booth, Isomi Miake-Lye, Jessica M. Beroes, and Paul G. Shekelle. "Mental Health Conditions Among Patients Seeking and Undergoing Bariatric Surgery: A Meta-Analysis." *JAMA* 315, no. 2 (Jan 12, 2016): 150-63 doi: 10.1001/18118 PMID: 26757464.

American Heart Association, *The New American Heart Association Cookbook, 25th Anniversary Edition,* 6th Ed. New York: Clarkson Potter Publishers, 2001.

Arthritis Foundation. "Weight Loss Benefits for Arthritis." Accessed March 13, 2021. Arthritis.org.

National Center for Home Food Preservation "General Freezing Information." Accessed April 5, 2021. NCHFP.UGA.edu.

Alley, Lynn. *The Gourmet Slow Cooker Simple and Sophisticated Meals from Around the World,* Berkeley: Ten Speed Press, 2003.

General Mills, Inc. *Betty Crocker's Do-Ahead Cookbook: 110 Easy Recipes That Are Ready When You Are!* Macmillan Publishing, 1994.

James, Meredith. "How Long Does Tofu Last" Accessed April 3, 2021. TofuBud.com.

O'Brien, P. E., A. Hindle, L. Brennan, S. Skinner, P. Burton, A. Smith, G. Crosthwaite, and W. Brown. "Long-Term Outcomes After Bariatric Surgery: a Systematic Review and Meta-analysis of Weight Loss at 10 or More Years for All Bariatric Procedures and a Single-Centre Review of 20-Year Outcomes After Adjustable Gastric Banding." *Obes Surg.* January 2019. 29, no. 1: 3–14 doi: 10.1007/s11695-018-3525-0. PMID: 30293134.

Public Education Committee. "Benefits of Weight Loss Surgery." Updated Sept. 2020 ASMBS.org.

Silvia Leite Faria, PhD; Mariane de Almeida Cardeal, MSci; and Orlando Pereira Faria, MD. "Protein Intake after Bariatric Surgery: A Review." *Bariatric Times* 17, no. 7 (July 1, 2020): 12-14.

Index

A

Almond Smoothie, Sweet Potato–, 103
Apples
  Apple-Cinnamon Flax Muffins, 51–52
  Cinnamon Apple "Pie," 150–151
Avocado Chocolate Mousse, 148

B

Banana-Oat Protein Balls, 76
Barbecue Chicken Tenders, 132
Bariatric surgery. *See also* Meal prepping
  about, 4–5
  dietary stages, 5–8
  lifestyle changes, 9–11
Batch cooking, 21
Beans
  Quinoa and Black Bean Bowl, 74–75
  Three-Bean Salad, 153–154
  Zesty Fava Beans, 110–111
Beef
  Low-Carb Meat Lasagna, 61–62
  Meat Loaf and Cauliflower Mash, 47–48
  Slow-Cooked Beef Stew, 120–121
  Steak and Veggie Stir-Fry, 145
  Zucchini Boats with Meat Sauce, 84–85
Beet Berry Protein Smoothie, 31
Berries
  Beet Berry Protein Smoothie, 31
  Blueberry Tofu Smoothie, 32
Bone Broth, 29
Bowls
  Egg Roll Bowl, 130–131
  Farro and Fruit Breakfast Bowl, 86–87
  Quinoa and Black Bean Bowl, 74–75
  Tropical Breakfast Bowl, 79–80
Broccoli, and Mozzarella Quiche,
    Crustless Tomato, 108–109
Broth, Bone, 29
Burritos, Low-Carb Breakfast, 112–113
Butternut Squash Soup, 125
Buttery Lemon Codfish, 143

C

Cabbage and Carrot Slaw, Crunchy, 157
Carrot Slaw, Crunchy Cabbage and, 157

Cauliflower
  Cauliflower Fried Rice with
    Shrimp, 135–136
  Cauliflower Tofu Puree, 36–37
  Creamy Chicken and
    Cauliflower Rice, 72–73
  Meat Loaf and Cauliflower Mash, 47–48
Cheese
  Chicken and Cheddar Chili, 59–60
  Chicken Cordon Bleu, 139–140
  Crustless Tomato, Broccoli, and
    Mozzarella Quiche, 108–109
  Low-Carb Breakfast Burritos, 112–113
  Shrimp Parmigiana, 137–138
Cherry Shake, Chocolate, 102
Chia Pudding, 105
Chicken
  Barbecue Chicken Tenders, 132
  Bone Broth, 29
  Cajun Chicken Sliders, 88–89
  Chicken and Cheddar Chili, 59–60
  Chicken Cordon Bleu, 139–140
  Chicken Pesto Roll-Ups, 141–142
  Chicken Tortilla Soup, 118–119
  Creamy Chicken and
    Cauliflower Rice, 72–73
  Fragrant Chicken Curry Stew, 126–127
  Saucy Chicken Meatballs, 63–64
  Slow Cooker Chicken Cacciatore, 70–71
  Spicy Chicken Salad, 158–159
Chocolate
  Avocado Chocolate Mousse, 148
  Chocolate Cherry Shake, 102
  Chocolate Peanut Butter Shake, 66
  Double Chocolate Hummus, 149
Cinnamon Apple "Pie," 150–151
Codfish, Buttery Lemon, 143
Curry Stew, Fragrant Chicken, 126–127

D

Dairy-free
  Barbecue Chicken Tenders, 132
  Cauliflower Fried Rice with
    Shrimp, 135–136
  Chocolate Cherry Shake, 102

Dairy-free (*continued*)
  Colorful Tofu Stir-Fry, 90–91
  Egg Drop Soup, 30
  Fragrant Chicken Curry Stew, 126–127
  Garlic and Ginger Teriyaki Pork, 133–134
  Overnight Oats, 65
  Red Lentil Mash, 38
  Saucy Chicken Meatballs, 63–64
  Slow-Cooked Beef Stew, 120–121
  Spicy Chicken Salad, 158–159
  Steak and Veggie Stir-Fry, 145
  Zesty Lemon Salmon Packets, 77–78
Desserts
  Avocado Chocolate Mousse, 148
  Cinnamon Apple "Pie," 150–151
  Double Chocolate Hummus, 149
  Mango Yogurt Pops, 152

E

Egg Roll Bowl, 130–131
Eggs
  Egg and Salmon Snacks, 92
  Egg Drop Soup, 30
  Low-Carb Breakfast Burritos, 112–113
  Veggie Egg Cups, 49
Equipment, 18–20
Exercise, 11

F

Farro and Fruit Breakfast Bowl, 86–87
Fish and seafood
  Buttery Lemon Codfish, 143
  Cauliflower Fried Rice with
    Shrimp, 135–136
  Egg and Salmon Snacks, 92
  Honey Salmon with Tangy
    Tzatziki Sauce, 144
  Lettuce-Wrap Shrimp Tacos with
    Chips and Guacamole, 93–94
  Salmon Cakes with Yogurt-
    Dill Sauce, 45–46
  Seafood Chowder, 122–123
  Shrimp Parmigiana, 137–138
  Zesty Lemon Salmon Packets, 77–78
5-ingredient
  Beet Berry Protein Smoothie, 31
  Blueberry Tofu Smoothie, 32
  Chia Pudding, 105
  Chocolate Cherry Shake, 102
  Chocolate Peanut Butter Shake, 66

  Mango Yogurt Pops, 152
  Peach Parfait, 39
  Tropical Protein Power Smoothie, 100
Flax Muffins, Apple-Cinnamon, 51–52
Freezing, 21
Fruit Breakfast Bowl, Farro and, 86–87

G

Garlic and Ginger Teriyaki Pork, 133–134
General diet (stage 4)
  about, 8
  Banana-Oat Protein Balls, 76
  Cajun Chicken Sliders, 88–89
  Chicken and Cheddar Chili, 59–60
  Colorful Tofu Stir-Fry, 90–91
  Creamy Chicken and
    Cauliflower Rice, 72–73
  Egg and Salmon Snacks, 92
  Farro and Fruit Breakfast Bowl, 86–87
  Lettuce-Wrap Shrimp Tacos with
    Chips and Guacamole, 93–94
  Low-Carb Meat Lasagna, 61–62
  meal plans, 56–59, 67–69, 81–83
  Overnight Oats, 65
  Quinoa and Black Bean Bowl, 74–75
  Saucy Chicken Meatballs, 63–64
  Slow Cooker Chicken Cacciatore, 70–71
  Tropical Breakfast Bowl, 79–80
  Zesty Lemon Salmon Packets, 77–78
  Zucchini Boats with Meat Sauce, 84–85
Ghrelin, 4, 10
Ginger Teriyaki Pork, Garlic and, 133–134
Gluten-free
  Avocado Chocolate Mousse, 148
  Banana-Oat Protein Balls, 76
  Barbecue Chicken Tenders, 132
  Beet Berry Protein Smoothie, 31
  Bone Broth, 29
  Buttery Lemon Codfish, 143
  Cajun Chicken Sliders, 88–89
  Cauliflower Tofu Puree, 36–37
  Chia Pudding, 105
  Chicken and Cheddar Chili, 59–60
  Chicken Pesto Roll-Ups, 141–142
  Chicken Tortilla Soup, 118–119
  Chocolate Peanut Butter Shake, 66
  Cinnamon Apple "Pie," 150–151
  Creamy Chicken and
    Cauliflower Rice, 72–73
  Crunchy Cabbage and Carrot Slaw, 157

Crustless Tomato, Broccoli, and
    Mozzarella Quiche, 108–109
Double Chocolate Hummus, 149
Easy Homemade Granola, 106–107
Egg and Salmon Snacks, 92
Egg Drop Soup, 30
Egg Roll Bowl, 130–131
Farro and Fruit Breakfast Bowl, 86–87
Flourless Protein Pancakes, 50
Green Goodness Smoothie, 101
Honey Salmon with Tangy
    Tzatziki Sauce, 144
Low-Carb Meat Lasagna, 61–62
Mango Yogurt Pops, 152
Overnight Oats, 65
Peach Parfait, 39
Quinoa and Black Bean Bowl, 74–75
Red Lentil Mash, 38
Savory Gazpacho Shake, 104
Spicy Chicken Salad, 158–159
Sweet Potato–Almond Smoothie, 103
Three-Bean Salad, 153–154
Tomato, Lentil, and Vegetable Stew, 124
Tropical Protein Power Smoothie, 100
Veggie Egg Cups, 49
Zesty Fava Beans, 110–111
Zesty Lemon Salmon Packets, 77–78
Zucchini Boats with Meat Sauce, 84–85
Granola, Easy Homemade, 106–107
Guacamole, Lettuce-Wrap Shrimp
    Tacos with Chips and, 93–94

H

Honey Salmon with Tangy
    Tzatziki Sauce, 144
Hormones, 4, 10
Hummus, Double Chocolate, 149
Hydration, 9

L

Lasagna, Low-Carb Meat, 61–62
Lemons
    Buttery Lemon Codfish, 143
    Zesty Lemon Salmon Packets, 77–78
Lentils
    Red Lentil Mash, 38
    Tomato, Lentil, and Vegetable Stew, 124
Lettuce-Wrap Shrimp Tacos with
    Chips and Guacamole, 93–94
Lifestyle changes, 9–11

Liquid diet (stage 1)
    about, 6
    Beet Berry Protein Smoothie, 31
    Blueberry Tofu Smoothie, 32
    Bone Broth, 29
    Butternut Squash Soup, 125
    Chocolate Cherry Shake, 102
    Egg Drop Soup, 30
    Mango Yogurt Pops, 152
    meal plan, 26–28
    Sweet Potato–Almond Smoothie, 103
    Tropical Protein Power Smoothie, 100

M

Mango Yogurt Pops, 152
Meal prepping
    about, 23
    benefits of, 14–16
    for families, 22
    general diet plans, 56–94
    liquid diet plan, 26–32
    principles of, 21–22
    puree diet plan, 33–40
    soft diet plan, 41–52
    steps, 16–18
Meatballs, Saucy Chicken, 63–64
Meat Loaf and Cauliflower Mash, 47–48
Muffins, Apple-Cinnamon Flax, 51–52
Mushrooms, Turkey-Stuffed, 155–156

N

Nut-free
    Apple-Cinnamon Flax Muffins, 51–52
    Barbecue Chicken Tenders, 132
    Beet Berry Protein Smoothie, 31
    Bone Broth, 29
    Buttery Lemon Codfish, 143
    Cauliflower Fried Rice with
        Shrimp, 135–136
    Cauliflower Tofu Puree, 36–37
    Chia Pudding, 105
    Chicken and Cheddar Chili, 59–60
    Chicken Cordon Bleu, 139–140
    Colorful Tofu Stir-Fry, 90–91
    Creamy Chicken and
        Cauliflower Rice, 72–73
    Crunchy Cabbage and Carrot Slaw, 157
    Crustless Tomato, Broccoli, and
        Mozzarella Quiche, 108–109
    Egg and Salmon Snacks, 92

Nut-free (*continued*)
Egg Drop Soup, 30
Egg Roll Bowl, 130–131
Farro and Fruit Breakfast Bowl, 86–87
Flourless Protein Pancakes, 50
French Onion Soup, 116–117
Garlic and Ginger Teriyaki Pork, 133–134
Green Goodness Smoothie, 101
Honey Salmon with Tangy
Tzatziki Sauce, 144
Low-Carb Breakfast Burritos, 112–113
Low-Carb Meat Lasagna, 61–62
Meat Loaf and Cauliflower Mash, 47–48
Peach Parfait, 39
Pumpkin Protein Pudding, 40
Quinoa and Black Bean Bowl, 74–75
Salmon Cakes with Yogurt-
Dill Sauce, 45–46
Saucy Chicken Meatballs, 63–64
Savory Gazpacho Shake, 104
Shrimp Parmigiana, 137–138
Slow-Cooked Beef Stew, 120–121
Slow Cooker Chicken Cacciatore, 70–71
Steak and Veggie Stir-Fry, 145
Three-Bean Salad, 153–154
Tomato, Lentil, and Vegetable Stew, 124
Turkey-Stuffed Mushrooms, 155–156
Veggie Egg Cups, 49
Zesty Lemon Salmon Packets, 77–78
Zucchini Boats with Meat Sauce, 84–85
Nutrition, 10–11

O

Oats
Banana-Oat Protein Balls, 76
Easy Homemade Granola, 106–107
Overnight Oats, 65
One pot/pan
Bone Broth, 29
Butternut Squash Soup, 125
Buttery Lemon Codfish, 143
Cauliflower Fried Rice with
Shrimp, 135–136
Chicken and Cheddar Chili, 59–60
Fragrant Chicken Curry Stew, 126–127
Garlic and Ginger Teriyaki Pork, 133–134
Seafood Chowder, 122–123
Steak and Veggie Stir-Fry, 145
Tomato, Lentil, and Vegetable Stew, 124
Onion Soup, French, 116–117

P

Pancakes, Flourless Protein, 50
Peach Parfait, 39
Peanut Butter Shake, Chocolate, 66
Pesto Roll-Ups, Chicken, 141–142
Pork, Garlic and Ginger Teriyaki, 133–134
Pre-op diet, 5–6
Proteins, 6–11
Puddings
Chia Pudding, 105
Pumpkin Protein Pudding, 40
Pumpkin Protein Pudding, 40
Puree diet (stage 2)
about, 7
Avocado Chocolate Mousse, 148
Cauliflower Tofu Puree, 36–37
Green Goodness Smoothie, 101
meal plan, 33–35
Peach Parfait, 39
Pumpkin Protein Pudding, 40
Red Lentil Mash, 38

Q

Quiche, Crustless Tomato, Broccoli,
and Mozzarella, 108–109
Quinoa
Quinoa and Black Bean Bowl, 74–75
Tropical Breakfast Bowl, 79–80

R

Recipes, about, 23
Reheating, 22

S

Salads
Crunchy Cabbage and Carrot Slaw, 157
Spicy Chicken Salad, 158–159
Three-Bean Salad, 153–154
Salmon
Egg and Salmon Snacks, 92
Honey Salmon with Tangy
Tzatziki Sauce, 144
Salmon Cakes with Yogurt-
Dill Sauce, 45–46
Zesty Lemon Salmon Packets, 77–78
Seafood. *See* Fish and seafood
Shakes. *See* Smoothies and shakes
Shrimp
Cauliflower Fried Rice with
Shrimp, 135–136

Lettuce-Wrap Shrimp Tacos with
    Chips and Guacamole, 93–94
Shrimp Parmigiana, 137–138
Smoothies and shakes
  Beet Berry Protein Smoothie, 31
  Blueberry Tofu Smoothie, 32
  Chocolate Cherry Shake, 102
  Chocolate Peanut Butter Shake, 66
  Green Goodness Smoothie, 101
  Savory Gazpacho Shake, 104
  Sweet Potato–Almond Smoothie, 103
  Tropical Protein Power Smoothie, 100
Snacks, 15
  Banana-Oat Protein Balls, 76
  Egg and Salmon Snacks, 92
Soft foods diet (stage 3)
  about, 7–8
  Apple-Cinnamon Flax Muffins, 51–52
  Buttery Lemon Codfish, 143
  Cinnamon Apple "Pie," 150–151
  Crustless Tomato, Broccoli, and
    Mozzarella Quiche, 108–109
  Flourless Protein Pancakes, 50
  meal plan, 41–44
  Meat Loaf and Cauliflower Mash, 47–48
  Salmon Cakes with Yogurt-
    Dill Sauce, 45–46
  Spicy Chicken Salad, 158–159
  Three-Bean Salad, 153–154
  Tomato, Lentil, and Vegetable Stew, 124
  Turkey-Stuffed Mushrooms, 155–156
  Veggie Egg Cups, 49
  Zesty Fava Beans, 110–111
Soups, stews, and chilis
  Butternut Squash Soup, 125
  Chicken and Cheddar Chili, 59–60
  Chicken Tortilla Soup, 118–119
  Egg Drop Soup, 30
  Fragrant Chicken Curry Stew, 126–127
  French Onion Soup, 116–117
  Seafood Chowder, 122–123
  Slow-Cooked Beef Stew, 120–121
  Tomato, Lentil, and Vegetable
    Stew, 124
Stage 1. See Liquid diet (stage 1)
Stage 2. See Puree diet (stage 2)
Stage 3. See Soft foods diet (stage 3)
Stage 4. See General diet (stage 4)
Steak and Veggie Stir-Fry, 145

Stir-fries
  Colorful Tofu Stir-Fry, 90–91
  Steak and Veggie Stir-Fry, 145
Storage containers, 19–20
Sweet Potato–Almond Smoothie, 103

T
Tacos with Chips and Guacamole,
    Lettuce-Wrap Shrimp, 93–94
Three-Bean Salad, 153–154
Tofu
  Blueberry Tofu Smoothie, 32
  Cauliflower Tofu Puree, 36–37
  Colorful Tofu Stir-Fry, 90–91
Tomatoes
  Crustless Tomato, Broccoli, and
    Mozzarella Quiche, 108–109
  Savory Gazpacho Shake, 104
  Tomato, Lentil, and Vegetable Stew, 124
Tortilla Soup, Chicken, 118–119
Turkey-Stuffed Mushrooms, 155–156
Tzatziki Sauce, Honey Salmon
    with Tangy, 144

U
Under 10
  Avocado Chocolate Mousse, 148
  Blueberry Tofu Smoothie, 32
  Chocolate Cherry Shake, 102
  Chocolate Peanut Butter Shake, 66
  Double Chocolate Hummus, 149
  Green Goodness Smoothie, 101
  Mango Yogurt Pops, 152
  Savory Gazpacho Shake, 104
  Sweet Potato–Almond Smoothie, 103
  Tropical Protein Power Smoothie, 100

V
Vegan
  Butternut Squash Soup, 125
  Quinoa and Black Bean Bowl, 74–75
  Red Lentil Mash, 38
  Three-Bean Salad, 153–154
  Tomato, Lentil, and Vegetable Stew, 124
  Zesty Fava Beans, 110–111
Vegetables. See also specific
  Steak and Veggie Stir-Fry, 145
  Tomato, Lentil, and Vegetable Stew, 124
  Tropical Breakfast Bowl, 79–80
  Veggie Egg Cups, 49

Vegetarian. *See also* Vegan
  Beet Berry Protein Smoothie, 31
  Chia Pudding, 105
  Chocolate Cherry Shake, 102
  Cinnamon Apple "Pie," 150–151
  Colorful Tofu Stir-Fry, 90–91
  Crustless Tomato, Broccoli, and
    Mozzarella Quiche, 108–109
  Double Chocolate Hummus, 149
  Easy Homemade Granola, 106–107
  Flourless Protein Pancakes, 50
  Green Goodness Smoothie, 101
  Mango Yogurt Pops, 152
  Peach Parfait, 39
  Pumpkin Protein Pudding, 40
  Savory Gazpacho Shake, 104
  Sweet Potato–Almond Smoothie, 103
  Tropical Protein Power Smoothie, 100
  Veggie Egg Cups, 49

W
Water, 9

Y
Yogurt
  Mango Yogurt Pops, 152
  Peach Parfait, 39
  Salmon Cakes with Yogurt-
    Dill Sauce, 45–46

Z
Zucchini Boats with Meat Sauce, 84–85

ACKNOWLEDGMENTS

First, I need to thank my mom, Maria. Without her I would never have had the confidence to pursue my master's in nutrition or write a book. Thank you for teaching me the importance of not giving up, working hard, and following my dreams.

My sweet boys, Daniel and Charles, who motivate me each day to work hard. May you always chase your dreams. And a special thank-you to all the boys at home, Michael too, for being my taste testers and giving me your unfiltered honest opinions; it certainly keeps me humble.

An extra-special thanks to my amazing man, my rock, Ron. I couldn't have done this without your support. I'm so grateful you kept me laughing on the long days and shopped for all the last-minute ingredients.

To my sister Maria and cousin Donna, for being on call while I was recipe testing or for last-minute ingredient questions.

To my patient-turned-dear-friend, Kelly. Your input and advice provided me with invaluable insight.

Thank you to all the patients who shared their journeys with me. A special thank-you to Alison, Chrissy, Jeena, and Karen for always being open and willing to accept even the toughest challenges. You inspire me daily.

And finally, to the Dr. Ferzli bariatric team I had the honor of working closely with for six years. It was a privilege to learn from you. Thank you again, Dr. Ferzli, Dr. Vulpe, Donna, Linda, Debbie, Kalista, Liz, Karen B., and Karen S.

ABOUT THE AUTHOR

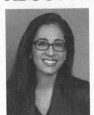

Andrea D'Oria has been a dietitian for 20 years. She received her master's degree in clinical nutrition from New York University in 2004 and has counseled more than 1,000 patients in weight management. It was in 2014 that she found her niche, working as the bariatric nutritionist for Dr. George Ferzli, a pioneer in laparoscopic surgery. In June 2019, Andrea started her virtual nutrition practice, Andrea D'Oria Nutrition. She is grateful to be able to help individuals achieve their health goals safely after surgery. Andrea lives in New Jersey and is a proud mom and often short-order cook for two young boys. She enjoys long bike rides, running, and summer days by the beach.